MEDICAL MALADY

MEDICAL MALADY
SURVIVAL IN A MINEFIELD OF MEDICAL MISTAKES

PRAD MITRA CHAUDHURI

PRADCO INC.

FIRST EDITION
PRADCO INC.
(Process Refining and Development Company Incorporated)

Medical Malady.
Survival in a minefield of medical mistakes.
A memoir of an unspoken yet important social issue of our times—medical mistakes.

Copyright © 2012 by Prad Mitra Chaudhuri.

All rights reserved under International and Pan-American Copyright Convention. No part of this work may be reproduced, stored or transmitted in any form or by any means—graphic, electronic or mechanical, including photocopying, recording, taping or information storage and retrieval systems—without the prior written permission of the writer and or the publisher (photocopying license is obtainable from Access Copyright 1-800-893-5777). The scanning, uploading and distribution of this book via the Internet or via any other means without the permission of the author and or the publisher is illegal and punishable by law. Please purchase only authorized electronic editions and do not participate in or encourage electronic piracy of copyrighted materials. Your support of the author's rights is appreciated.

Published in Canada by:
PRADCO INC.
5100 Erin Mills Pkwy
PO Box 53032 ERIN MILLS
Mississauga, Ontario, Canada L5M 5H7

www.medicalmaladies.com

Certificate of Registration: The United States Copyright Office,
June 4, 2012. Prad Mitra Chaudhuri.
Certificate of Registration of Copyright, Canadian Intellectual Property Office,
April 5, 2012. Prad Chaudhuri

Library and Archives Canada Cataloguing in Publication

Chaudhuri, Prad, 1944-, author
Medical malady : survival in a minefield of medical
mistakes / Prad Chaudhuri.

ISBN 978-0-9919404-1-7 (pbk.)

1. Chaudhuri, Prad, 1944- --Health. 2. Medical errors.
I. Title.

R729.8.C53 2013   362.1092   C2013-905368-9
ISBN 978-0-9919404-2-4 (ebook)

Cover photograph: Prad Chaudhuri
Cover design: Team PRADCO Inc.
Text design and formatting: Tania Craan

Printed and bound in Canada: Friesens

For Nihar,
Gale, Bobby, Monica and Neil,
and those who lose their lives by the thousands, each day, around the world,
and the victims of collateral damage, who suffer in silence without a voice,
and the diligent and dedicated doctors, nurses,
and other health care professionals who help the disabled
victims recover and return to their families,
and the taxpayers who ultimately bear the burden of
preventable medical mistakes:
medical maladies.

This book was written from the vantage point of one person: the author. It contains graphic description of events as they unfolded, some of which may be disturbing to some readers.

CONTENTS

PROLOGUE 1

PART 1: **MONTREAL, 1994** 3

PART 2: **CALGARY, 1994** 55

PART 3: **THUNDER BAY, 2003** 83

PART 4: **MONTREAL, 1995** 111

PART 5: **TORONTO, 1996** 145

PART 6: **SASKATOON, 1998** 195

PART 7: **PITTSBURGH, 2000** 245

AUTHOR'S NOTE 264

END NOTES 266

ABBREVIATIONS 269

LIST OF PEOPLE 271

ACKNOWLEDGEMENT 277

PROLOGUE

JUNE 30, 1994. Gale and I call it Day Zero, the day when all things changed, the day from which we count everything else. The late-night phone call sent us running from Calgary to Montreal, and when we arrived, we found Bobby—our first-born—lying on an ICU bed in a twilight between the living and the dead, deep in a coma. We stood there staring at him, confused, terrified. How could this be? What could have happened? Yes, Bobby was anaphylactic to peanuts, but he was a doctor, not a child. He knew what to do in the event of poisoning. He was careful to the extreme regarding the ingredients in food that touched his lips.

We were certain he wouldn't have poisoned himself. Why would he? He was about to start a residency at a prominent hospital. He had everything to look forward to. Still, this was the impression that we were being given—that he had poisoned himself. But would he really have come to the hospital if he had? None of it made any sense. Especially this: When Bobby arrived at the hospital, they should have known what to do. Did they? If so, how had he ended up in a coma?

The woman, the only other person who had been with him when it all happened, wasn't much help. She was uncooperative—hostile, even. She seemed to be hiding something. Over those first few days—then weeks, then months, then years—our confusion and grief turned into a search for the truth. We haven't found all the answers, but the ones we have found may astound you.

Years later, when the time came to reveal those answers, I was

MEDICAL MALADY

forewarned: If I went public, the worst would happen. It did, but not immediately. Shortly after the story broke in the *Globe and Mail*, the telephone rang in my office. The call display disclosed the caller's location: the Calgary Room—one of several namesake meeting rooms down the hallway past two sets of double doors. Yet the caller instructed me to go to the Halifax Room. It was the closest one to the HR department, as I recall. That was where the hatchet man would ask you to leave your keys and credit card before escorting you out the door, minus your laptop computer and cellular phone.

The hatchet man, with four others around the table, handed me a letter as I walked in. Then, minutes later, a strange reversal: They rescinded and asked me to stay on. This reversal of their decision allowed me to retire nine months later, with a golden handshake, a pension and a complete set of golf clubs.

That was October, Y2K. I left Canada to work in Pittsburgh's research park, resigned to spend the sunset of my career in the green hills of Monroeville. The loonie was sixty-two cents then. I could've toughed it out, kept quiet, gone on with life. But the compulsion to tell the whole story myself, not merely the slice of it that had already gone public through a narrowly focused newspaper article, brought me back to my tiny vineyard outside of Toronto. Otherwise you wouldn't be reading what happened on that horrible day. The events of June 30, 1994 started us down the road toward a terrifying diagnosis: decorticate. The prognosis? "The chance for recovery to a meaningful functional state: nil."

This is the story of that day, that diagnosis and everything that followed. It is the story of what can go wrong in the murky medical–legal world and why. It is a story that may make you rethink your relationship with your own healthcare. Most of all, it is a story about things you should know.

PART 1:
MONTREAL, 1994

1

MIDNIGHT CALL

JUNE 30, 1994. "I am afraid Bobby had another peanut episode," Jen announced over the telephone from Montreal. It was 11:40 P.M. in Calgary, two hours behind. Gale was preparing for bed, and I was running the kitchen tap for a drink of water. Mon, nineteen, and Neilly, twelve, were in bed, as was grandmother Nihar—in poor health.

"Where is he?" A chill went up my spine as I tried to stay calm. Gale had picked up the extension upstairs, and her scream pierced the night. "Oh, no… my God…no…what happened?"

"He's in ICU…we had Chinese take-out…Dr. Zan will call back," Jen said, sounding eager to end the conversation.

Bobby had called earlier, at 10 P.M. He'd arrived in Montreal late that afternoon following a five-day drive from Calgary. He was ready to start his neurology residency at the same general hospital the following morning. Jen had tagged along; initially, she wasn't supposed to be on the trip. Her call was unexpected, her tone unfamiliar and her message both cryptic and horrific.

"What do you mean, Chinese take-out?" I asked. "He told me he had Swiss Chalet! We will be there on the first flight out. Don't throw away any of the Chinese food." I couldn't believe Bobby would order in Chinese food, let alone with nuts in it! I wanted to see it for myself. He was a doctor, not a child, and he was well aware of his allergy.

Jen's voice switched gears. "You…you don't have to come. After all, where, where would you stay? My dad will be coming to fix the furniture in the apartment."

PART 1: MONTREAL, 1994

I struggled to take in what Jen was saying. Her father, Al—an ex-Franciscan monk about my age, and as bald and bulky as I looked at fifty—didn't travel; he lived with his girls in a modest house in northwest Calgary. He spoke in a low voice, rarely raising his eyes from the floor in conversations, and gave away handmade trinkets. Bobby had received a couple of them since meeting Jen at a debate tournament. She was younger, in St. Mary's High, when Bobby was majoring in biochemistry at the University of Calgary.

Blue-eyed, straight blond hair, pale white skin on a flat anatomy, Jen was highly intelligent. She kept her thin mouth, sporting a chipped front tooth, mostly shut. She'd met Bobby on the rebound—shortly after her boyfriend had left for Halifax. At the time, she was attempting to balance the affluent lifestyle of her single mother and the simple lifestyle of her artistic father. While Al endeared himself to Bobby with his simplicity and honesty, Jen became attached like a vine to a tree.

Al going to Montreal to assemble Bobby's IKEA dining table—the only piece of furniture that remained unopened in a box, our graduation present to our firstborn on his way to becoming a neurologist—felt strange, ominous. Bobby and I had rented the spacious apartment and furnished it just ten days before; I'd paid the rent to kick-start his career and life in Montreal.

MY TREMBLING HAND SCRIBBLED, "3:30 A.M.," in the open Hilroy logbook I used for work, when Dr. Zan called, followed by: "Needed CPR 5–10 seconds, and stopped breathing."

With the telephone number, name and coordinates of the ICU chief noted, I called back ten minutes later to verify the particulars. The voice on the other end of the line assured me that Zan would call back when things settled.

Zan did call back. "Sixty percent oxygen right side [of chest affected], vomited, on life support [system]... paralysis, still on paralyzing [agent]..." She was called away again. Things didn't settle.

In the background, Gale muttered, "Told him so many times to

MEDICAL MALADY

stay in Montreal, not to fly back with Dad, not to take the car…" She hadn't wanted Bobby to drive from Calgary to Montreal, but to remain there following the apartment hunt and rely on public transit. His car was old, and to her, unreliable. Now, that was the least of our problems.

THE TELEPHONE RANG AGAIN AT 5:07 A.M., just as I'd started to doze off. The logbook was open on the dresser by the telephone. The pen rested where I'd stopped writing. I knelt on the floor and resumed scribbling as fast as Zan could exhale words. "Bizarre movement of extremities, not waking up, seizure damage in brain. Dr. Panis neurologist, not a good sign."

Sounding utterly perplexed by the symptoms, Zan hung up. I held the receiver in my hand, fully awake now. The nightmare was real.

I got up in haste to go to the ensuite bathroom, steps away. The sudden rise caused a momentary shortage of oxygen to my brain. I could hear Gale yelling as she tried to pull me up by the hand. I could feel the pain of mangled eyeglasses on my face.

I gathered my senses and got on the telephone with the airline. "Thank God Mom is here to look after the kids so I can go with you," Gale said, not for the first time. She was accustomed to packing my bags in a hurry for my frequent business travels as an engineering specialist, a process troubleshooter. Gale grabbed whatever she could for herself and shoved everything into one green Samsonite on wheels.

"Don't worry about a thing here—bring Bobby home." Nihar's words carried the confidence of her seventy-five years. I pressed a fifty-dollar bill into Mon's hand, gave her a hug and whispered, "Look after Neilly and Gramma." Her brown eyes welled. Neilly stood speechless. I reached for him, pulled him close, and said, "Listen to Gramma." He nodded, and we left.

DARK CLOUDS ROILED in our minds despite the sun-drenched Alberta morning as we made our way to the airport, about forty-five minutes from our Oakridge Estates neighborhood. The cabbie attempted small conversations in a thick Nigerian accent; I'd had many rides with him.

PART 1: MONTREAL, 1994

He chatted away, but soon gave up after hearing nothing more than "Uh-huh." There were no words between Gale and me—just unspoken anxiety.

Thin traffic gave us an hour and three-quarters to spare following the purchase of two full-fare tickets, and the luggage and security checks. It was Canada Day, and the Air Canada lounge was closed until 10 A.M. That left us roaming aimlessly, and then gravitating toward Tim Hortons, which Bobby normally avoided but for a large cup of coffee; his immune system would hysterically release histamine if it were exposed to the proteins in nuts—an occasional ingredient in muffins, cookies or chocolates. The process could choke him to death in minutes, by wrinkling smooth muscles and dilating blood vessels. Although Bobby carried an EpiPen—a self-administered antidote against poisoning—at all times, he always avoided pastries for fear of cross-contamination. His vigilance worked. He'd remained free of peanut poisoning until February 1992, when the med-school cafeteria served skewered beef with—unbeknownst to him—crushed peanuts. That incident brought home a hard lesson: He could trust, but he had to verify ingredients, every time.

Our large coffee cups were empty by boarding time, and a myriad of questions jangled in our minds. One tormented us more than the others: How had this happened? Was it ingredients or something else?

2

PARADOX

JUNE 30, 1994 IS ETCHED IN MY BONES and will remain there until their remains are tucked away in an urn or spread over the vines by the rows of Rose of Sharon I tend. It wasn't a typical memorable day—like a birthday or an anniversary—and yet I count each day from that date. Since then, no one and nothing can be trusted, unvetted, unscanned.

Twelve hundred and forty days from Day Zero, on November 17, 1997, a group of lawyers—huddled in the opulent boardroom of a large law firm, then known as Bennett Jones Verchere, on the 45th floor of the Bankers Hall East in downtown Calgary—took part in an examination for discovery. The subject was Jen—one of the key defendants in the suit we'd brought against all concerned with the events of and following June 30, 1994. Jen was the only other person in Bobby's apartment when it all began. She had the answers; we were sure of it—answers we desperately needed, to make sense of everything that had happened. Jen came prepared with Roon—her lawyer—and an eagerly waiting psychiatrist, outside the boardroom. The psychiatrist also happened to be Jen's mother.

Our lawyer pitched questions from his laptop. The pace was slow and easygoing, even friendly, to make Jen comfortable. At times, however, it could be rapid-fire, to cut through the bungle and expose thorny points.

Bill: Did the two of you ever live together?[1]
Jen: No.

PART 1: MONTREAL, 1994

Bill: Was it your intention to live together in Montreal?

Jen: No. I was going out to Montreal to do an elective at the Children's Hospital there, and also for a holiday before I started residency. I'd be coming back to Calgary after the elective.

Bill: How long were you going to do your elective there for?

Jen: I think it was only a two-week elective. I was going to be back to Calgary sometime I think in July.

Bill: Were you aware of his problem with anaphylaxis?

Jen: Yes.

Bill: And that was prior to going with him to Montreal on June 30, 1994?

Jen: Yes.

Bill: Did you understand that his anaphylactic reaction could potentially be fatal?

Jen: That's what he told me.

Bill: But you had no reason to doubt that, I assume?

Jen: No.

Bill: Now, amongst the food that was in the containers when you arrived back at the apartment, were there these dumplings in peanut sauce or not?

Jen: No.

Bill: Was there anything, then, that had nuts in it in the bag of food that came back to the apartment, to your knowledge?

Jen: Not that I know of.

The voluminous transcript arrived at our home via courier a few days later. Gale sucked up the contents like a sponge. That's how she was when it came to books, newspapers or magazines dropped in our mailbox at Oakfern Crescent, nestled in southwest Calgary.

Before our three kids were born, Gale had taught school, but she gladly gave it up to raise them. Motherhood had trumped her career and she found it hard to image an alternative. I clearly remember a kitchen conversation she had with Bobby shortly after he had started med school, prior to the cafeteria skewered-beef incident in 1992.

"It's awful; she abandoned her children," Gale said, referring to Jen's mother Nan. She watched Bobby gulp down his dinner, a quick bite before he'd return to the Health Sciences Centre. She was ruthlessly critical of a mother whose children appeared neglected in any way, especially if she thought that to be the mother's fault. However, she was always eager to forgive the shortcomings of the kids.

"Nan didn't abandon her children; she divorced Al for irreconcilable differences," Bobby replied, mouth full. "Glass of milk, please!"

"And who raised them?" Gale asked, probing further.

"Al did, from the time Jen and her younger sister were toddlers."

Gale poured a glass of milk. "How did Jen get that chipped front tooth?" With the presumption of neglect, she pressed on, passing the glass.

"She fell from her father's workbench when she was little." Bobby stood up to leave.

Gale rested her case. She had little respect for Nan—though Nan had become a psychiatrist after leaving her husband and her kids—but she did have a soft spot for Jen, one of the "abandoned children."

AS DIFFICULT AS IT WAS to accept some of the answers in the transcript, Gale was ready to give Jen the benefit of the doubt. I wasn't, not since the call in the middle of night, and certainly not since Day 2.

"'Not that I know of'—then where did the nuts come from?" I asked. "'A holiday before I started residency' suggests she was already a doctor. But she was just a first-year medical student!"

Answers eluded me. Bobby had been meticulously vigilant in avoiding exposure to peanuts. Everyone associated with him knew that—he'd made sure of it since February 1992.

For anaphylactics, poisoning by peanuts would be far worse than poisoning by anthrax. Bobby'd said it himself. "[The] first symptom [of peanut poisoning] would be an impending sense of doom . . . tingling around the lips and tongue, the shortness of breath, then hoarseness and then dizziness and then loss of consciousness."

Bobby's loss of consciousness on Day Zero made no sense. And the

PART 1: MONTREAL, 1994

eventual diagnosis—decorticate?—absurd. That one word—which means "without the brain function that makes one human"—changed everything that I had known to be truthful and true. That trust-busting word shook the foundations of professionalism to the core. It was like a quake that exposed an ugly paradigm that was beyond my comprehension, beyond the reality I'd known before that fateful day.

I prune the overgrown vines and shudder. Rose of Sharon in full bloom sways in the changing wind.

3

EMIRATE

MONTREAL. THE CITY WAS FULL OF GRIDLOCKS—the luggage conveyor at Dorval airport, knotted traffic on Metropolitan Boulevard, and the creaky elevator at the hospital that stopped at every floor, though no one could be seen or heard around 5 P.M. on this particular Friday. The ICU was on the third floor. Two right turns along an eerie hallway led us to the entrance, through an imposing stainless steel door recessed to the right. I left our rollaway luggage in the adjacent waiting room before picking up the red telephone for permission to enter. "We are Bobby's parents. Okay to come in?" Gale attempted to peer between the door panels, ready to push.

The nurse held the telephone for a minute and checked with someone before clearing our entry. The door wasn't locked. Jen hurried past without a word, a clergy close behind. The sight of him shook us both—*my God, is it too late?* I glanced at them as Gale hesitated momentarily before moving ahead. *Were they reading the last rites?* Jen looked nervous, yet somehow defiant as she went out of the ICU.

The beds in the row on the left were all occupied; some on the right were as well. Each bed could be curtained off from the floor to the ceiling tracks and made into a rectangular, white-fabric cubicle, leaving ample space between the rows. Parental instinct pointed us to Bobby's bed—the one in the far left corner with the open curtain. Gale got closer, stroked his hair. Holding back tears, she whispered, "Mom and Dad are here to take you home, Bobby." I had no idea if he could hear her.

PART 1: MONTREAL, 1994

With the curiosity of a process troubleshooter, I nervously scrutinized our son, who was barely recognizable through the tangle of tubes. An eight-millimeter endotracheal (ET) tube plunged into his mouth and branched into a Y. Its right arm was attached to a ventilator, which was helping him breathe. Its left arm was hooked up to a bag—a large, stiff balloon tied to the oxygen supply. This would allow the nurse to squeeze air into his lungs if the machine failed. A nasogastric (NG) tube stuck into one of his nostrils was held firmly in place with surgical tape that ran under it and crisscrossed at the tip of his nose. Its job was to expel stomach contents. The other end was inserted into a trap that led to a wall-suction. Bobby's cheeks—in fact, his entire face—was puffy; his eyes were motionless and almost shut. The left eye was peeking slightly—the way it used to twenty-two-and-a-half years before, when he was in his crib, just after Gale would put him to bed and turn off his bedroom lights. That Christmas baby, our firstborn, was now completely unresponsive, suspended like a fly in a web.

Everything in the cubicle was movable or adjustable. The bed could be raised or lowered, tilted or rolled. From the oval ceiling track above Bobby's bed hung three hangers on rollers—two supported four dangling bags of fluids, and the other supported only two. Each bag was unmistakably marked: KCl, NaCl, glucose and such. The monitor read his heart rate, blood pressure and oxygen saturation. A catheter drained into a measuring device that led to a container. Medications sat on a table on wheels on the right side of the bed, the ventilator on the left.

Bobby appeared asleep, yet awake; his eyelids didn't react to my hand on his forehead—the only place I could touch him. "Can you hear me, Bobby?" I repeated after Gale, "Can you squeeze my hand? We are here to take you home." I had the distinct sensation that he was relieved.

I turned to the attending nurse, Fay, who was middle-aged, slender and efficient—very much guarded. Her answers to my questions were short and to the point.

"Do you know who the attending was when Bobby arrived in the ICU?"

"It was Joan," replied Fay, with reluctant consideration.

Dr. Gord, an ICU fellow, was nearby. She wasn't talkative either, but seemed approachable.

No sooner had we exchanged words than a man, who appeard to be four-hundred pounds of flesh on a six-foot frame, stormed out of an office a couple of beds away and began hurling bursts of words between puffs of breath. "Hi, I am Dr. Spa; I am the director of the ICU. I run this place."

"Bobby's our son—" I said, pointing at the bed next to us.

"I know." His deep, irritated voice cut me off in mid-sentence. "The rule is you must leave when the nurses work on him and ask for permission to get back in."

"What happened to Bobby?" I asked anxiously, as he straightened his appearance.

"He had an anaphylactic shock and a massive aspiration."

A prolonged pause followed, as if the communication line had gone dead. An aspiration? Spa offered no explanation, how Bobby's stomach contents had found their way into his lungs, clogging them up as aspirates would. Was this why his stomach was hooked up to the wall suction? The need for answers overtook my grief.

"Thank you," I said, facing the barricade of his folded arms.

Gale's tears dried up in the desert of compassion. The swish of rubbing fabrics broke the silence. His disheveled enormity, draped in a hanging shirttail, waddled off in the direction of its appearance. To underscore our first encounter with the supreme power of the closed system, the nurse kicked us out. She was about to suction Bobby's ET tube.

NIHAR'S NETWORKING soon brought Gupta, a family friend, to the ICU. He was visiting his sister-in-law in Montreal. "Are you hungry?" he asked.

We weren't, not for food, but certainly for some support. We walked

PART 1: MONTREAL, 1994

with him to Swiss Chalet—a peanut-free restaurant on Côte-des-Neiges, north of Côte-Ste.-Catherine—where Bobby and I had eaten supper just over a week ago. It was where I thought Bobby had gone the night before. Gupta was a busy man, a professor at the University of Calgary Business School from a young age. His sister-in-law, Ratna, was the dean of the Faculty of Education at McGill University. She was about to leave for New York, but he assured us that she would come and see us on her return.

"What could possibly have gone wrong?" asked Gupta, as we were about to leave the restaurant following the hasty visit. The answer to his question would've been easier if Bobby wasn't a doctor, or if didn't have a car, or if his apartment wasn't close to the very hospital at which he was to start work at daybreak. But none of it made sense—not the Chinese food, not the take-out, not whatever had caused the aspiration. "Thankfully, he was able to get to the hospital to seek help," Gupta said.

I answered his earlier question with one of my own: "What caused him to become comatose?"

7:30 P.M. THAT QUESTION COMPELLED US to visit Bobby's apartment after a short stop by his bedside. We walked out of the ICU into the waiting room and came face to face with Jen. I needed the keys. She wasn't ready to hand them over, but agreed to show us where the car was parked. I followed her and Gale to the elevator. Jen took the long way around, avoiding the ER and exiting through the main entrance. We made our way to Bobby's gray 1987 Pontiac, across the street from the ER.

The car was parked on Côte-Ste.-Catherine, a little more than half a block southeast of Côte-des-Neiges. I asked again for the keys, this time to put the luggage into the trunk so we wouldn't have to lug it around. She hesitated but eventually complied. I unlocked the doors to the passenger side to let Gale in, and ushered Jen to the back seat. I knew exactly how to get to the Rockhill apartment. I had been in and out multiple times to rent and furnish it.

MEDICAL MALADY

Jen said little as we drove. When we asked what had happened, she mumbled in a measured monotone, "It's too painful for me to talk about it." She was clearly playing the victim. Odd, since Bobby was the one in the hospital.

The car hadn't steered well since Bobby had climbed over the traffic island at Glenmore Landing Shopping Centre on 90th Avenue in Calgary; he had called me to get it dislodged. I took a right turn on Côte-des-Neiges and right again, past the sixth traffic light and into the surface parking lot of the building complex. A swing left around the parked cars and a short right took us to the down-slope of the underground garage. The roll-up door wouldn't open without a key, either on the way in or out. The complex decorated the skyline with several highrises, in an attractive setting that backed onto Saint Joseph's Oratory, facing a large cemetery across Côte-des-Neiges. The apartment balcony overlooked a fashionable clubhouse and a swimming pool. Brian Mulroney, then prime minister of Canada, had apparently met his wife, Mila, here when they were young. The rental agent probably repeated the story a thousand times to entice prospective young tenants.

Floors 10, 11 and 12, went by as the elevator ascended and clunked at 14—missing 13. Jen followed us into the apartment but remained out of sight by the closet in the narrow hallway. To the right of us was a bathroom and a single bedroom around the corner; to the left was a spacious dining room. The kitchen was off the dining room, ahead on the left. The hardwood floor and hot water heat had been two of the selling features for the allergy-prone tenant. The two IKEA chairs that Bobby and I had assembled—signing their undersides—remained under the chandelier, undisturbed. The large, flat box of the unassembled dining table rested on the wall to the left. We headed for the opening that led into the kitchen. The room was small. The fridge was to the right, the stove to the left and the sink beyond it. On the countertop stood two wine glasses, empty save for the dregs of red wine. The dishes were spotless, bearing no sign of the claimed Chinese takeout. Bobby's telephone, the one and only in the apartment, rested on the kitchen countertop, just where we'd left it a week before.

PART 1: MONTREAL, 1994

"Where is the Chinese food?" Gale and I hollered in chorus.

"I threw the garbage out." Still out of sight, Jen yelled her answer back.

"But the garbage is all here, in the cardboard box, just the way it was when Bobby and I left last week!"

"I couldn't bear the sight of the Chinese food."

"When did you throw it out? I told you not to!"

"I came to the apartment before you arrived."

"Where did you throw it out?"

"Don't know."

She held her ground. Her answers to our questions were short and ready—like those of a debater in cross-examination. An old debate judge, I chose to give her the benefit of the doubt. Getting Bobby back to consciousness was all that mattered.

Our search—through the living room, the walkout balcony, and the bedroom to the left of the bathroom—uncovered no sign of any Chinese food. The blue sheets and the matching comforter, on a bed frame that Bobby and I had assembled and placed the mattress over, were new. A shower curtain that hadn't been there before was hung, and the shower had been used before our arrival.

Restless, Jen had us take her back to the hospital. We returned to the apartment around 10:00; Gale resumed her search. I entered the bathroom, opened the cupboard and discovered four little red Benadryl tablets missing from a leaf of twelve. Gale found an empty EpiPen syringe—marked 0.3 ml/inj, October 12, 1993—in the dining room closet.

"Where are the brand new EpiPens I gave him just before he left Calgary?" she exclaimed. The old pen had bought him time—around 15 minutes—to get medical attention.

Looking for the EpiPens, I discovered Bobby's wide-open knapsack on the floor by the foot of the bed, his Life Alert® bracelet and wristwatch beside it.

"Strange," I said. He always kept his bracelet and watch on him, but he'd take them off and place them next to him when he'd sleep.

It was a habit I had observed during many trips with Bobby since his graduation from high school.

Leaving the old EpiPen, his watch and the Life Alert on the floor by the frenzied knapsack, seemed utterly out of character.

"You think Bobby was sleeping when it happened?" Gale asked, puzzled.

Instinctively, I murmured, "Yes." Any other possibility seemed absurd.

JULY 2. BOBBY SPENT THE NIGHT ON A NORCURON DRIP—a short-acting neuromuscular blocking agent derived from snake venom. We spent the night on chairs in the waiting room. Like paralyzed prey, he had been unable to respond for the nearly twenty-five hours that had elapsed since our arrival. Much later, we were told that Norcuron masked the visual signs of his seizures. Without aggressive anticonvulsant treatment, an electrical storm was raging in his brain.

Spa took him off Norcuron in the morning and put him on Ativan. It was a belated anticonvulsant treatment, but an anticonvulsant treatment nevertheless.

A technologist used a portable X-ray machine on the patient in the next bed. Bobby was within range of radiation, yet no protective covering was offered. I muttered aloud, "Someday I might want grandchildren." The tech apologized and left.

Gurgling noises could be heard from Bobby's throat, signalling a buildup of mucus in his airway. A nurse began to suction, triggering coughs, gags and shakes. His still body jumped in progression with a rusty whistling sound of increasing intensity. When the noise got nastier, we were told to leave.

Fatigued and famished, we agonized in the waiting room, craving any word of assurance. Elaine, Ratna's young research assistant, appeared like an angel through the dismal doorway, coffee and muffins in hand. She delivered them with hugs and a voice filled with concern. "What have they said happened to Bobby?" she asked. Ratna had called Elaine from New York and sent her to help.

PART 1: MONTREAL, 1994

"He was deprived of oxygen," I replied, regaining my voice in the warmth of coffee and kindness.

"My God! How did that happen?"

"That's what we are here to find out."

Calm prevailed when the nurse let us back in. She was taking Bobby's temperature. No fever. She put him on Phenobarbital—the drug of choice for treating seizures in infants.

My engineering instinct went into overdrive. I observed the monitor, jotting down signs of wakefulness—a slight twitch of the left toe—and making notes as to when the ABP (an arithmetic average of systolic and diastolic blood pressures) took a nosedive below 50, triggering a piercing alarm. The nurse looked as worried as Gale and I. She put on a brave face but showed us the door.

When we were allowed to return, the slight twitch in Bobby's left toe had grown into a prolonged, vigorous shake, as if a storm that had begun slowly was taking the shape of a hurricane. By nightfall, we were introduced to the rudiments of neurology: myoclonus—an involuntary burst of nerve impulses at fixed frequency—and seizures—a movement that would start with rhythmic twitches, progress to a steady state, and then subside.

Nearing the 48-hour mark, Bobby opened his right eye. Perhaps repeated pleas to squeeze our hands had reached the center of his brain, or perhaps our nightly vigil, together with the anticonvulsant and the withdrawal of Norcuron, had produced results. The vigil, however, ended abruptly. Out of the blue, and in a voice a decibel or two higher than normal, Spa banned us from spending the nights in the waiting room. Gale and I looked at each other, perplexed. We obeyed his decree and hoped for change. The last thing we wanted was to rock the boat. The vigil became restricted to nightly telephone calls from the Rockhill apartment.

JULY 3. The day began with sun on our faces and pain in our backs—from lumpy sleeping bags. We shared a superstition: Bobby would return to his bed, and soon, if we kept it unoccupied and clean. Not since we'd moved into our first home in Sarnia had we slept on hardwood floors. Bobby had been around eighteen months old then. He would sit on my stomach, play horsey and lie face down on my chest to doze off, cradle cap in view—the first sign of an allergic child, Gale would diagnose after reading Spock. He had become sensitive to the birch trees located on either side of our spacious front yard. I'd replaced them with apple and cherry trees—fitting for a neighborhood that had been an orchard before the builder had turned it into family homes.

It was nearly 8 A.M. We hurried off to the ICU, arriving as Dr. Panis, the weekend neurologist, was conducting a full neurological examination. At around noon, he delivered positive news: Bobby had moved his eyes in direct light—indicating brain stem function—and retracted his fingers on induced pain. The neurologist returned in the evening for another set of examinations. While Bobby's eyes started to react, myoclonic actions—restricted to the eyelids and the left toe—had appeared for short durations. "These are encouraging signs," Panis assured. "If he can keep up this momentum, things should get better."

The nurse repositioned Bobby from his right side to his left. He reacted with a jump in BP, with coughs, and by opening his mouth. She decreased his Ativan. "Hopefully, this will increase his wakefulness," she said, as his blood pressure fell back down. The high ABP alarm was set at 115, the low at 50. The nurse would acknowledge the alarm, on either side of the range, and seemed ready to take action. Gale, on the other hand, watched in stunned silence.

ONE OF THE YOUNG DOCTORS who had treated Bobby in the ER showed up at 7:00 in the evening and volunteered to tell us what had happened.

"He walked into the hospital [by himself] at 11:00–11:05 P.M," said Dr. Koh. "He told the nurse, 'I can't breathe, I can't breathe. I am anaphylactic to nuts. I was intubated before; I think I had nuts.' The nurses gave him epinephrine, tried to put an intravenous—IV—line in. He was already thrashing around at this point. His heart and pulse

PART 1: MONTREAL, 1994

stopped for 30 seconds max, and the doctors started CPR. By this time his airway had become very constricted.

"Three ER doctors tried to intubate him," Koh continued. "He vomited and some of the vomit went into his lungs, which complicated air going into his lungs. His [blood oxygen] saturation was between 30% and 60% for about an hour before the vomit and mucus could be suctioned off and saturation could be brought up to the 90%+ level"—which is normal. They tried to get the O_2 level from 30% to 60% and then from 60% to 90% in steps. If Bobby had gone to the ER an hour later—past shift change—he would have had only one doctor.

Koh seemed believable. I had no reason to doubt his story, but I took notes anyway, just as I did when Fay advised us to look for signs of irritability and chewing on the ET tube. She didn't mention these as signs of seizures, but the staff seemed to be afraid of it without actually uttering the word. The Ativan drip was stopped, and anti-seizure drugs—Dilantin and Phenobarb—were introduced.

MONDAY MORNING. THE ICU RESIDENT, Dr. Sull, announced that Bobby's EEG didn't show myoclonic (seizure) activity, but that the brain activity had slowed compared to the previous tracing. The brain wasn't flat but slowed, he reiterated. This news didn't stop Bobby from opening his eyes at 12:57 P.M.—on request. Our excitement couldn't be contained. Spa looked up in disbelief, approached the bed and ordered Bobby to open his eyes. No response. Spa's massive hands landed hard on Bobby's sternum, shaking the unresponsive body. Still no response. He left without a word.

Dr. Scho, a bearded, yarmulke-clad neurologist with a nearly imperceptible nervous twitch, appeared in the afternoon and examined Bobby for half an hour. "Bobby might wake up and smile in a couple of days, or take a month to come around," he explained in a low-key methodical manner. "He will not be Karen Quinlan—his brain stem functions and all his reflexes are intact. Whether Bobby will be like Bobby is difficult to say. It is too early. He's had a very bad insult to his brain."

MEDICAL MALADY

Insult or not, early in the evening, Bobby tried to move his left hand as I repeated the Mulroney story loud enough for everyone to hear. He moved his head toward us. His left eye opened wide on request, the right only slightly. He moved his shoulder and arm. Was this an indication of the sleep–wake cycle that one of the nurses had been talking about? If so, this was clearly a wake cycle. Nurse Katrina washed Bobby's hair and shaved the parts of his face that were free of tapes and tubes. He looked better, drooling a bit, moving a little, but there was scant strength in his grip. He wasn't squeezing my hands on request, although the Dilantin and Phenobarb seemed to have started to work.

The head nurse and the respiratory therapist were ready to suction. Bobby was perspiring; his BP was up, as was his pulse—signs of another wake cycle. After fifteen minutes, we were allowed back in. He seemed to look at us through the slight opening of his right eye. I held his right hand; he couldn't squeeze my hand but he did try to move his shoulder and arm. Gale and I sat still, holding hands, as he fell back into unfathomable sleep. At times there were movements of his loosely shut eyes, perhaps it was REM, that left us wondering and waiting—for him to wake up from his world of dreams.

No one in the McGill neurology program at the MNI—Montreal Neurological Institute—knew what had happened to Bobby. I had left a message for the program director, Dr. Francis, to inform him, but I also hoped Francis might rescue him from the cave of coma. After all, this was the best neuro facility in the country—the reason Bobby had ranked this neurology residency first on his list.

Dr. Scho's words—"Bobby will not be Karen Quinlan"—resonated in our minds as the first-year internal medicine rotation at the hospital, JGH, went into full swing—with one less doctor in the ward and one more patient in intensive care.

4

MEAL

TORONTO, 2006. GALE DUSTS OFF VOLUMES of transcript notes in our collection, to take a peek at the ones that intrigue her the most—like the story in Jen's deposition. I bring in branches of Vitis vinifera and leave them on the round kitchen table to extract the leaves. Spiders and earwigs scamper out of the twisted vines and drop to the floor. Our lives do not revolve around the burning questions any more, but the questions burn nevertheless, especially around bold discrepancies.

Bill: Now, when you went to the unit clerk, you were given his wallet. Is that what you said?

Jen: They had his wallet.

Bill: And that was minutes after your arrival at the hospital that you picked up his wallet?

Jen: It was shortly after. I can't remember if I took his things or whether they kept his things, but they had his wallet with them and we were going through, looking for his address and insurance number and that kind of thing.

Bill: And that was within minutes of your arrival at the hospital. Correct?

Jen: Yes. It was shortly after—I wasn't looking at a watch or a clock. I had gone into the patient area, was there for less than a minute, and then was ushered out to the unit clerk.

Bill: Are you sure that you picked up the wallet or not?

Roon: I don't think she said she picked it up.

MEDICAL MALADY

Jen: I don't remember whether I took it or whether they kept it.
Roon: I don't think she said she picked it up.
Bill: I just wanted to understand what her evidence was.
Jen: They had the wallet there.
Bill: And did you pick it up at that time?
Jen: I think we both at different times had it in our hands and were looking through it. I don't remember if afterwards I was given his things to keep or whether they kept them.
Bill: Did you have any other discussions with the unit clerk or anybody else about getting his valuables back subsequent to that?
Jen: I don't remember any.
Bill: Can we go to page 469—466 of my record, 469 of yours. I mean the Montreal chart. You'll see that the time recorded in terms of the picking up of valuables was 1:30 in the morning.
Jen: Mm-hmm.
Bill: Do you have any explanation for the discrepancy between what you're describing and this note?
Jen: I don't think there is a discrepancy. I said I didn't remember whether I had taken the wallet at the time that I was talking to the unit clerk down in emergency. And so, when we were going through this stuff down below, that was shortly after I'd come in. I don't remember signing the record for the valuables actually ever.
Bill: But that is your signature on that document, is it?
Jen: Yeah.

I catch a glimpse of the page Gale is reading. "Roon had no idea Jen had picked up Bobby's wallet from the ICU before calling us," I say as I chase and squash the bugs on the floor. She closes the binder and yells, "Not only that, she had picked up Bobby's gold-rimmed glasses, high school graduation ring and gold chain as well." Gale's recollection is usually perfect, while I rely mostly on my diary.

PART 1: MONTREAL, 1994

AL AND BARB—NAN'S SISTER—ARRIVED IN THE hospital at midnight the day after our arrival in Montreal. They had checked into the Royal Terrace Hotel. Nan was beyond voice contact on a hiking trail somewhere on Vancouver Island with her Irish boyfriend. Barb came instead, although her husband in Victoria was seriously ill.

Shortly after their arrival, we let Jen take Al and Barb into the apartment. Jen zeroed in on a bundle of laundry she'd presumably left in the closet. "These are Bobby's sheets and towels," she declared. She put the bundle through the basement laundromat at 1:30 A.M. and took it with her to the hotel. The sheets and towels were returned to Gale a few days later; we left them in the suitcase, unopened to this day.

Gale discovered a crumpled customer copy of a MasterCard bill the following morning, after Jen returned Bobby's wallet, presumably at the urging of her aunt or her father. It showed a payment of $30.71 to "La Perle de Szechuan 0413-0407." The receipt was hand written, without any date or address on it. On the bill was Bobby's signature and staple marks where a cash register receipt had once been attached. That receipt could have cleared up some unanswered questions.

Nan appeared the following night, with her entourage—Jen, Al and Barb—all smiles. She approached Bobby's bed and exclaimed in short, high-pitched spasms, "Hi, this is Dr. B. I am here." The spectacle ended with her saying, "Ooh, I can have him now," as she departed for the hotel in holiday spirit, leaving us befuddled. Her entourage followed. Jen appeared relieved to have her mother on the scene.

JULY 5. BACK FROM NEW YORK, Ratna called early in the morning and woke our crashed bodies and crushed minds. The telephone calls from friends and relatives hadn't stopped all night long; the news of Bobby's coma had spread with electronic speed. I scrambled to call Dr. Cuttrell, the post-graduate Year 1 (PGY-1) coordinator at the McGill University medical residency program. She had no knowledge of Bobby's situation. "What happened to Bobby?" she asked.

Later, at the hospital, one of the three ER doctors from Day

Zero—Dr. Rose—dropped in. His curiosity and concern seemed to transcend one doctor treating another. He claimed he had come into the ER following Bobby's collapse.

As the days passed, the relatives of some of the ICU patients became more than nodding acquaintances. Molly's husband, a divorce lawyer, had had a heart bypass operation. He was to have returned home in a day or two, but that was weeks before. Something went haywire and she wasn't being told what. In her sixties, without support, she resorted to talking to herself—no food, no drink and no sleep. Gale's urging brought her to the cafeteria for supper. She had the last withered slice of what had once been a pizza. I asked the woman at the counter for a glass of milk. "Today is meat day," she growled. No one drinks milk on meat day!

"I'm sorry," I said, not being familiar with such custom at any hospital in the past.

3:40 P.M. Bobby squeezed my hand ever so slightly and repeated the action on request. His grip wasn't strong. He was breathing more on his own now, about 18 or 19 breaths a minute, while the ventilator did 10. He had started making progress once the Norcuron was withdrawn and anticonvulsants introduced. He moved his left leg, bending at the knee, and tried moving his left hand. His heart rate jumped up to 119. He seemed to startle at my calling out, "Bob . . .Bob."

Joan relieved Natalie at shift change. I knew nearly all the ICU nurses by this time, except Joan—the one who had seen Bobby when he arrived at the ICU from the ER on July 1, somewhere between 1:00 and 1:30 A.M. I thanked her for her care during the wee hours of that morning; she deserved the compliment. In her version of events, Bobby had come to the hospital ER on Day Zero between 11:00 and 11:05 P.M. and remained there until 1:30 A.M. the following morning—until stable. Between 5:30 and 6:00 A.M. in the ICU, his blood pressure had dropped drastically and he became "convulsive and unstable." This seemed to corroborate my notes.

PART 1: MONTREAL, 1994

JULY 6. NAN'S ARRIVAL SEEMED TO BRING about a dramatic change in Jen's behavior, and in that of the hospital staff. A surrogate family now encircled Bobby—parents, aunt, and a pretend spouse. Jen crouched ever closer, nearly covering Bobby's face as she read a book to him in an unintelligible rapid chant. The night nurse reported that mother and daughter were visiting past midnight:

Bill: And insofar as you were reading to him, did that seem to quiet him in any way?
Jen: I can't be sure. It quieted me.
Bill: Did anyone tell you that there were no seizures present in Bobby? In other words, that they'd ruled out epilepsy?
Jen: I don't remember them saying this. I really tried to stay away from the medical parts of what was going on.

Dr. Friedman, a third-year Internal Medicine resident, saw Bobby during nightshift. His fever was down but there was no neurological improvement. His left thumb, toe, eyes and chin were shaking. The neurologist was called in. The nurse advised us to buy a pair of high-top basketball shoes to support Bobby's ankles and prevent foot drop—the inability to flex feet backward that comes from lying in bed with little or no voluntary movement. Bobby was breathing on his own, although the respirator remained hooked up.

At 12:30 P.M., Dr. Scho examined Bobby for a prolonged period and emerged with a lengthy explanation. "His brain is busy seizing, which is why he is not responding and recovering. He will be given a large shot of Phenobarbital and Dilantin to stop the seizures. The Phenobarb will keep him quiet until the end of the week."

The distinction between myoclonus and seizures was becoming clearer, as was the fact that it would be impossible for Bobby to wake up if he continued to seize. By 1 P.M., he'd been given an extra dose of Dilantin, along with Phenobarbital. By 2:40 P.M., the seizures had stopped and our hope was renewed.

Not for long though, as trouble brewed elsewhere. Shortly thereafter, Nan and Jen appeared in the ICU. The door to Spa's office closed behind them as we watched from the open cubicle. Soon, Spa emerged from the office, and boomed, "Bobby ate food clearly marked peanuts in 1992!"

"How do you know?" I asked.

"I talked to the Foothills doctor."

The Foothills doctor? Foothills was a hospital near our home in Calgary. I wondered if Nan was the doctor he'd referred to. Clearly, it was an attempt to shift the blame. But why?

AN ELDERLY VOLUNTEER, Elaine, arrived in the waiting room. She was pleasant but stoic, compassionate yet detached, but more importantly, she displayed no bias.

When Elaine returned the following day, I asked her to look up the address of the restaurant Jen claimed she and Bobby had gone to. Various versions of the Chinese food story had gotten around: one from Jen, the others from the doctors and nurses. All probably came from the same source, at different times—before Nan's arrival and after. They ate in the restaurant, ate out of the restaurant, took food to the apartment, and so on. Elaine found La Perle de Szechuan at 3515-25 Lacombe Avenue.

Gale returned from a visit with Ratna and we set out to search for a pair of high-top shoes. The black canvas basketball shoes with white trim and white cotton socks fit perfectly, but were ridiculously out of place in the ICU. Nevertheless, they provided a lighter moment amidst the adversity, a mixture of smiles and tears.

I called Mon mid-afternoon to bring her up-to-date, as we did every day. She held back her good news until the end of the conversation. "Something I ought to tell you," she said. "I got into U of A Med School." I had had no doubt that she would. Mon was a straight A student with an impressive array of accomplishments—a silent worker.

"Should I accept or postpone?" she asked.

PART 1: MONTREAL, 1994

I couldn't agree to her postponing. "Go ahead, accept," I said firmly. "Your life must move forward, and not be put on hold like ours."

5:30 P.M. BOBBY WAS DEEP IN A SLEEP CYCLE when Gale and I ventured out to La Perle de Szechuan on Lacombe, not far from the hospital. The side street was part of an ethnically diverse working-class neighborhood. For one new to Montreal, it was a difficult street to find, and it proved nearly impossible to spot the restaurant's green signboard. Faced with two entrances, we chose the main one, to the left by the cash register. No other customers were visible in the dining room. The one and only waiter ushered us to a table, served two glasses of water and produced an eat-in menu.

"Do you have a take-out menu?" I asked.

He promptly handed us a folded green pamphlet, showing the take-out specials—a variety of combinations at different prices.

Mr. Tam—part owner of the restaurant, forty-something, taller than an average man of Chinese heritage, slightly balding—remembered Bobby and Jen from Thursday, June 30, between 8 and 9 P.M.

"He ordered package B," he told us in perfect English. "The only take-out that had the Hunan dumplings in hot sauce."

"What kind of sauce?" I asked.

"Peanut butter sauce," he said, explaining that it was a mix of peanut butter and Hunan spices.

Gale and I ordered package B, eat-in. Tam told us that he'd just opened the restaurant the Saturday before last Thursday. "Bobby and Jen had gone for the pick-up food because they got a 10% discount," elaborated Tam. "He [Bobby] called the restaurant and asked for the dumplings that were not in the bag when they returned to the apartment. The driver went to "deliver the dumplings, but left out the rice." Tam had called MasterCard to get Bobby's telephone number, to tell him that rice was coming. As soon as the driver returned, Tam said he gave the rice to the driver and the driver went back to the apartment. Bobby apparently opened the door, accepted the rice and invited the man in for a cup of coffee.

The more Tam spoke, the more his story sounded fictitious, far-fetched. If the dumplings had been left out, it must have been because Bobby had known that the sauce was poison to him. He wouldn't have called the restaurant. Besides, there seemed to be too many transactions in Tam's story, and calling MasterCard for customer information simply wasn't credible. At the time, Gale and I were left perplexed.

Tam's story seemed concocted. It became clear when we discovered, down the road, that Nan had visited the restaurant before we did, without our knowledge. Details came much later:

Bill: Now, did you ever go to the Chinese food restaurant after June 30th, '94?
Jen: No.
Bill: Did you go with your mother? Did your mother go?
Jen: My mom went.
Bill: What did she find out when she went?
Jen: I think she went just because she wanted to see where it happened. I don't know what she asked there. I think when we talked about it, all that she did was just went and saw where it was and looked at the menu.
Bill: Did she ever discover who it was who talked to you?
Jen: I don't remember her saying so.
Bill: Could you make inquiries of her and determine what she learned on the occasion of her visit to the restaurant, please, and advise me through your counsel.

Just what Nan was up to, surruptitiousy visiting the restaurant, and lingering in the ICU—with no relation to us, or to Bobby—all of a sudden seemed to have a purpose. A purpose hidden from us at the time, the facts about the Chinese food—had there been any—brought into the apartment on Day Zero, that we had been attempting to uncover.

Back in the restaurant, Gale and I noticed that the MasterCard

PART 1: MONTREAL, 1994

receipt and the prices on the takeout menu didn't match—with or without the discount and or taxes, and least of all for Package 'B.' Had they eaten in the restaurant, not in the apartment? Bobby's allergic reaction was instantaneous, a fact that Tam had no way of knowing.

The dumpling sauce was spicy, hot to the touch. A strong peanut butter odor permeated the restaurant as the food was brought in. I shook my head. Bobby couldn't tolerate that smell, not since childhood. If the dumplings had been brought into his apartment, it was without his knowledge. However, there was no evidence of Chinese food in the place. How, then, had the poison gotten there? Worse, how had it gotten into his mouth?

5

ALIBI

A CRISP SUMMER MORNING; the city stood still. Our walk to the hospital was quiet and took longer than normal. We passed a bearded old man, standing barefoot and motionless, blending into the backdrop of St. Joseph's Oratory. Out of habit, I squeezed the tiny knob on my obsolete Texas Instrument digital watch that I'd bought in Houston. July 7, 1994, it read. Our meeting with Brenda at the hospital accounting department wasn't until 9 A.M. When we arrived, she was ready with the out-of-province claims form needed for the hospital to collect $610 per day from Alberta healthcare for the ICU bed. We left her satisfied with the paperwork. The occupant of that bed, Bobby, was being prepped for a CT scan.

That morning, he was consumed with seizures on his left side—the side that moved when stimulated. The neurologist was in. The nurse had administered Pentothal—a short-acting anesthetic—which triggered a sharp drop in Bobby's blood pressure that scared us stiff. Our eyes were fixed to the monitor as he was transported to the radiology floor.

Within the hour, Bobby was back. The combined action of Ativan, Phenobarb, Dilantin and Pentothal had a dramatic effect in lowering his BP. When it wore off, he appeared stable, and we went searching for Dr. Scho, eager for the scan results.

No brain swelling, he said. The CT scan was normal. He wouldn't ask for an EEG until after the weekend. Bobby might not need a tracheotomy—a required step for prolonged ventilator assistance. He

PART 1: MONTREAL, 1994

would likely come out of coma before the procedure was necessary. Scho, however, would keep Bobby at higher-than-normal doses of Phenobarb and Dilantin to keep him seizure free. "Seizures have a tendency to perpetuate," he said.

The tranquil sleep cycle ended with a yawn in the afternoon. Bobby opened his eyes, tried to move his left leg and squeezed my hand with his. The effort sped up his heart rate. As excited as Gale and I were, the resident on duty was not convinced that the actions were purposeful.

Periods of sleep and wakefulness went on.

Someone had called Jen when Bobby was being moved to radiology. She appeared but soon left, showing little interest. It was another indication of the strange world we found ourselves in—a world where we, his parents, weren't called or consulted in the ICU, nor invited to attend closed-door meetings. Yet I was asked to sign papers involving the hospital claims.

JULY 8. BOBBY HAD BEEN PLAGUED with seizures through the night. Overstimulation triggering convulsions emerged as a point of concern. The nurse filled us in. Jen had paraded as a "resident," visiting past midnight and disrupting his sleep cycles. The nurse resorted to Pentothal push, 100 mg at a time. Another seizure spell began as the morning dose wore off, prompting another dose. The technologist prepared to hook up an EEG machine, sending us off to the waiting room.

As we waited, a white-haired man extended his hand to introduce himself. There was warmth in his handshake and empathy in his voice. This was Jack Antel, chairman of the MNI neurology program, the man who'd interviewed Bobby for the neuro-residency position. He'd already met with Scho and observed Bobby. He noticed some voluntary and some involuntary motions. The longer Bobby took to wake up, he warned, the poorer the prognosis and the poorer his chance of a full recovery.

The MNI's interest seemed to add vigor to the treatment of Bobby's seizures. The neurologist moved the Dilantin target to 80, and a nurse administered 500 mg over and above the regular dose. The constant seizures required the use of a mouthpiece to prevent Bobby from biting into the ET tube. The mouthpiece had caused a horrible sore on his lower lip. It had become swollen, chapped and red. The nurse administered ointment, eye drops and mouth freshener.

A physiotherapist brought in a therapeutic bed that was less prone to cause bedsores. Late in the afternoon, in sleep cycle, Bobby looked comfortable. The nurse overheard the neurologist saying that the EEG showed a slight improvement. She seemed sanguine of recovery, and genuinely concerned about Bobby's odds of stumbling and falling when "he stepped out of coma." She recommended a pair of sturdier high-top shoes for better ankle support, and pronto, we ventured out again to face the soaring Montreal temperature and humidity—following relentless rain. The nearby Rockland Shopping Centre was a welcome change from the bleak confinement of the ICU—virtually cut off from the rest of the world, where kosher cafeteria food was the norm, and no one drank milk on a meat day. When we returned with a spiffy pair of fine white leather high-tops with grassy green trim and a new pair of white socks, a minor tremor remained.

Jen's best friend and Dan, Bobby's med school classmate, arrived from Calgary at her invitation, an unwelcome intrusion during our difficult time. The presence of any unnecessary visitors raised our fear of infection and additional seizures. The night that followed was as dreadful as the one before. Eleven Pentothal pushes, the nurse informed us, and yet the seizing continued into morning. A new anticonvulsant—Tegretol—was infused into Bobby's NG tube.

The crowd seemed to embolden Jen, and they visited the apartment for her personal belongings. Gale took pride in showing them Bobby's meticulous and cautious arranging of the kitchen cupboards—with spices, utensils and food that would allow him to avoid eating out. Why, she asked, would they go out to a Szechuan restaurant? Jen stormed out of the kitchen and out of the apartment.

LATER IN THE EVENING, Dan stretched out on a sofa in the waiting room, eyes closed, mouth open. A year before, he and Bobby had completed a month-long medical elective at the Mayo Clinic in Minnesota. I woke him up to ask if Bobby had had close calls with peanuts in his company. They'd shared a hotel room and had eaten all their meals out. Dan would've known if Bobby had ever been cavalier with his affliction. He shook his head from side to side. North American cooked food generally had no peanuts, barring chocolate bars and cookies, which Bobby avoided.

How Bobby happened to ingest peanuts on Day Zero remained a mystery. Al was to leave Montreal early the following morning. Gale and I saw our last opportunity to ask Jen, in front of her father, just what had transpired at that fateful moment. I was in no mood to accept, "It's too painful to talk about it," the excuse she'd used prior to her mother's arrival. Since then, it had become, "I've already told you many times." Nan would then jump up to interrupt with, "You're interrogating!"

The entourage arrived in the family waiting room at 8:45 P.M. I asked the families to remain and the rest to step outside so Jen could once again recount the events leading up to the trip to the ER. "We all need to hear the same story, once and for all," I pleaded.

Nan and Jen exchanged glances. Jen took a deep breath and started confidently. "Bobby and I went to the apartment after we picked up the Chinese take-out. I found some of the dishes were missing, and I asked Bobby to call the restaurant. Bobby picked up the phone and called the restaurant." It seemed as if Jen had anticipated this moment, and had prepared for it.

"Then you called," she said, pointing at me but as usual, not making eye contact. "Bobby picked up the phone. I was setting up the sheet on the floor when two more dishes came. The delivery person was either Timmy or Henry.

"The second time, one of the boys came and delivered the dumplings and rice.

"I was reading a cookbook, and Bobby took one of the dumplings and swallowed it. I said, oops, Bob, it has peanut sauce.

"We looked for the EpiPen; Bobby injected himself in the apartment. I drove Bobby to the emergency, dropped him off and went to park the car. While I was driving, Bobby took another shot of EpiPen."

MEDICAL MALADY

Al looked uneasy. "I thought Bobby drove himself to the hospital," he said.

Jen lost her composure. "I wasn't proud to admit that I didn't drive him to the hospital," she shot back. Strength in numbers had made it possible for her to battle the truth this far. Suddenly, though, the can of deception had popped open.

Gale, who'd never said a harsh word to anyone, couldn't contain her feelings. "Liar!"

My frustration bubbled to the surface. "You . . . you weren't even in the car!" Jen, a medical student, had let an anaphylactic—who could pass out on the road, a likelihood that she'd known since 1992—drive; she didn't call 911. All seemed utterly unbelievable. It was getting late; Jen's best friend and Dan had left already, and Al's flight was at 7:30 in the morning. I shook his hand to say goodbye. He pulled me closer, gave me a hug and said he was sorry for what had happened.

6

ALARM BELL

I LOOKED DOWN INTO THE BASEMENT from the top of the stairs. Bobby was lifting a heavy carton of books from a stack of used cardboard boxes.

"Do you want help?" I asked, as I watched him come up the stairs, walk through the passage—between the foyer and the steps to the kitchen on the right—and take a step down on the left into the attached garage, through the open side door.

"No, thanks," he said as he proceeded to load the trunk of his Pontiac. "I can manage."

It was around 10 A.M., June 25, 1994. He'd packed the boxes meticulously with his med school books, a favorite childhood blue-and-white rubber dog, Rolf,—allergies kept him from owning a real one—and a large pink Dino the dinosaur he'd won at the Calgary Stampede. An excess of beer, pop and irregular hours in his final year of med school had left his stomach protruding over his belt. Packing was a chore he hadn't had much experience with, although we had moved cross country since he was born. He was puffing.

"Did you get some film for your camera?" I asked. He had packed my Pentax SLR for the trip.

"I forgot. Would you buy me some?"

Bobby would overspend his budget and then beg us to buy things for him. Gale and I took him to London Drugs on MacLeod Trail, a short jaunt from Oakridge.

"Why's Jen going with you?" Gale asked. Jen's tagging along was a last-minute change of plans. She'd had Nan arrange a temporary two-week elective in short order. Bobby was going to pick her up from her father's house on the way out of town.

"Jen said she'll share the travel cost."

"Are you committed to this relationship?"

"No, we're just friends." Sitting comfortably in the back seat, Bobby continued in a serious tone. "I don't believe in long-distance relationships. I will be doing a residency in Montreal for the next six years and she'll be a medical student in Calgary for the next three. Who knows who I'll meet? This will be a goodbye trip."

We returned home around noon. About to leave, Bobby gave us a hug. My last words were, "Break a leg; don't kill yourself." It was cliché, but that's what I said, verbatim. He drove off, leaving me with a trail of thoughts.

During his first two years of med school, Bobby had lived at home, and had started to date Jen, an aspiring marine biologist at the time, before she'd decided to apply for med school. Since they met, he'd often been invited to either her father's house or her mother's. The twice-divorced Nan had held frequent parties for the young residents.

Insecure in her relationship, Jen would occasionally call our home in near panic and ask, "Is Bobby there? Where, where is Bobby?"

I would say, "Well, didn't you check the Bach Centre?" The Bach Centre was next to a large open area in the University of Calgary Health Sciences Building—a hangout for girls from the main campus looking to meet medical students.

"Yes, but he isn't there!"

"He might be at Dan's apartment watching hockey." Dan's apartment was Bobby's "escape," a place to watch hockey, play video games or get into a game of poker.

She would hang up in a hurry to find him. I found out later that Jen hadn't been into hockey, but she hung around the group nevertheless, remaining quiet without taking part in conversations. If they played poker, she would join in.

PART 1: MONTREAL, 1994

JULY 10. THE LOW ABP ALARM SHRIEKED. Concerned, I called the nurse. The hospital provided one-on-one care for critical-care patients, but not this time; the nurse seemed to be attending another patient. The doctors and nurses went into action as fear engendered paralysis in us. The BP stabilized within 10 minutes; meanwhile, all the ICU doctors were by the bedside.

Scho examined Bobby following rounds at 9:00 A.M., but left without speaking to us. Bobby had been seizing, and the seizures accelerated past 9:40 A.M., when Pentothal was pushed again. The medication didn't seem to treat the root cause of the seizures; it merely masked Bobby's movements and triggered the unwelcome consequence of lowering his blood pressure. The numbers improved by 11:14 A.M., but that didn't stop us from wondering how many patients met their end this way.

Dr. Crow, approachable, second in command in the ICU, came by to tell us that all Bobby's drug dosages had been changed. There was no indication of who had ordered the change. A continuous Pentothal drip was started intravenously and Valproic Acid was added via the NG tube. If he seized, even more Pentothal was pushed. Dilantin and Phenobarb were administered in higher dosages. The plan was to keep him well sedated and "quiet" until the doctors could evaluate him next.

The weather improved in Montreal, but the days weren't any brighter. Now in a drug-induced coma, Bobby's progress stalled. He was moving his hands, startling or having myoclonic jerks, but he was free of seizure movements. His BP remained unstable, but thankfully above the low-alarm point. Bobby's hands and feet were cold, his right hand swollen from the IV line and the cuff. The swelling in his lips had subsided a bit, although his stomach was distended from lack of motility. Still, he looked peaceful. The ICU nurses ran out of places to put the IV, and a new femoral line was put in. His kidneys were functioning well, seemingly not bothered by the low BP. Although he had the ability to breathe by himself, he was hooked up to the ventilator. The ICU staff wanted control of his airway—anesthetics depressed breathing.

MEDICAL MALADY

The nurses were used to us by now, and didn't kick us out as often. They were better at handling the patient, as we were in handling the bedside stress: watch the monitors, watch Bobby and pray in silence. An occasional alarm would go off around us, jolting us to attention. With the receptive nurses, we could often identify the problem and offer a solution. With the others, we remained quiet observers.

JULY 11. THE MNI'S CONTINUED INTEREST SEEMED to be keeping Bobby alive. They had been visiting, and I had been asking them for help in whatever way possible: from analytical support in titrating his blood Dilantin level to come up within therapeutic range, which was held up for analytical delays, to transferring Bobby to their facility. Dr. Francis assured us that if he recovered fully, or close to it, Bobby could be on medical leave and get back to work at any time.

Suggestions for ways to wake up Bobby poured in: let him listen to the current news on radio, play his favorite music—Rush, Revelation and Sting; read his favorite childhood books—Gordon Korman and Star Wars; let him smell a perfume he was familiar with but not allergic to. All, however, proved futile. The continued anesthetics kept the coma patient in a coma.

Jen's best friend and Dan waited patiently by the red phone, seeking clearance from the ICU staff to see Bobby before their flight to Calgary. I approached and asked them to contact the media, to start a citywide prayer service in Calgary. A complaint from Jen brought Spa out. "You are not letting them into the ICU to say goodbye. You are not the gate keeper here!"

He ushered Dan and the friend in. This revelation came later:

Jen: So at that point I think Dr. Spa talked to Bob's parents and was actually quite angry with them.
Bill: And, so, you continued to visit?
Jen: I said that I wanted to go home that night and not push the issue. Dr. Spa insisted that I stay. Bob's parents were not in charge; he was.

PART 1: MONTREAL, 1994

Bill: And do you recall when it was that you had that confrontation with the parents?
Jen: No.

The side rails were down as the visitors left. Bobby's leg was over the edge of the bed, the needle-areas were bleeding and no nurses were around. We called for help and the IV lines were adjusted and the needles repositioned. Before they left, the visitors were apparently given some news: Bobby had reached the fatal and final stage of status epilepticus.

Bill: Did you ever hear from Dr. Panis or somebody else that they'd diagnosed a condition called burst suppression syndrome?[2]
Jen: No.
Bill: How early in the piece [goings-on] was it that you got the impression that there was a nihilistic or grim prognosis for Bobby?
Jen: I think it had been building up to Dr. Spa's discussions, so even though it was a terrible shock to hear it from him actually said, it was something that I think they'd been trying to build up to.

Dan and Jen's friend returned to Calgary and held a wake for Bobby with their friends. One of them took on the task of planting a tree in Israel in Bobby's name.

7

TRANSITION POINT

ELEVEN DAYS PASSED. Bobby remained in the ICU on his back, motionless. Parts of his body were puffy, edematous. "They all swell up like this," Fay said. The ET tube couldn't bother him now—he remained completely consumed by the drug-induced coma. Infection became an added enemy; hospitals by nature harbor germs resistant to common antibiotics. Drawing frequent blood samples was routine, but the nurse had failed to get one in the last set of tries; another attempt was in progress. She gave up on his arms and began poking his ankles.

Bobby neither moved nor flinched as the nurse inserted needles into his pale white skin full of bruises from the repeated attempts to find a vein—in vain. Fay finished putting in a femoral line. The blood pressure machine read 120/62; the cuff was turned off. Pin-cushioned in both arms and legs, Bobby nevertheless seemed stable.

The evening shift brought Denise, a black, middle-aged nurse. Her compassion matched her large motherly frame. Bobby's diastolic pressure plummeted to 39. I whispered, "Look! I am scared." She gently removed his pillow to lower his head, allowing gravity to assist the blood flow to his brain—an extra measure of protection I hadn't seen done before. The O_2 saturation on the monitor was lower but within range. Denise turned around and squeezed me in a big hug.

JULY 12. THEY SWITCHED TO SALT to control Bobby's BP. His entire right hand became grossly swollen; his face puffier. The neurologist

PART 1: MONTREAL, 1994

walked in and said, "Perfect." He asked the nurse to reduce Pentothal by half, in steps. Once weaned, Bobby opened his eyes. No tremors. His eyes quivered and squinted a bit, and then closed when Fay suctioned him. Nobody kicked us out anymore for suctioning.

The nurse asked me to sign a consent form—for a tracheotomy and the administration of anesthesia, although Bobby was being anesthetized already and consent had been neither sought nor signed.

"Who would be the surgeon?" I pressed.

"Dr. Spa."

The thought of those massive hands that had nearly crushed Bobby's sternum began to weigh on mine. "Any dexterity left in those hands?"

Gale whispered, "Maybe a resident will do the work."

Dr. Gord had already ordered the increase in the anesthetic—presumably to prep Bobby for surgery. He became abysmally motionless as the Pentothal peaked. All other medications were raised as well. Dr. Scho vowed to take him off Pentothal the next day, regardless, and ordered a full EEG. If Bobby continued to seize, Scho admitted, he didn't know what to do next.

5:30 P.M. REPAIRS WERE IN PROGRESS in the waiting room, so patient families were sitting on benches in the area across from the stainless steel doors. Nan walked in, anxious, carrying a beige woven handbag of clicking bottles of whisky—clearly visible, clearly out of place. Spa ushered Nan and Jen into his office and closed the door, not long after we were allowed in to sit by Bobby's bedside.

They emerged shortly.

"If Bobby is to get better he should have done so by now," he barked. "Chances are that he won't make it."

Clearly referring to my efforts to get help from the MNI, he warned, "Don't try to go to the end of this world to get a cure for him. Patients like Bobby seize, seize, seize and die."

The words hit their target in asymptotic intensity. Gale broke down in despair. Convinced that a comatose patient could indeed hear, I got closer, and in a whisp of a voice spoke into Bobby's ear. "Prove the pumpkin wrong, Bobby. Prove him wrong. I won't give up on you, even if everyone else does."

Gale waited until the women departed, carrying the now-empty handbag. Choking back tears, she got the words out. "We want to take Bobby home to Calgary; we want him close to home."

Spa considered it for a moment and replied, "I will talk to Dr. Sand in the morning."

"Don't give up on Bobby, even if you think there is a one-in-a-million chance for him to get better," I pleaded from the floor.

"I won't unless his heart stops." His words echoed off the walls as he walked away.

6:10 P.M. BOBBY OPENED HIS EYES and made a face that looked like a smile as his systolic pressure migrated below 90. The nurse added saline to the IV line and his BP crept up to 100. She suctioned his stomach and gave a shot of Gravol for signs of nausea. Stomach settled, he appeared to be listening. Very alert, his eyes were open, looking at the empty ceiling, and he chewed on his tube. His heart rate and BP jumped and the rhythmic shakes resumed. Another bolus of Pentothal knocked the symptoms flat on the bed.

JULY 13. WE WENT LOOKING FOR A NEURO UPDATE at ten in the morning; Scho was in his office. It didn't take long to consult with him and return to the ICU. In shock and horror, we saw that Bobby's BP had plummeted to 67/39. No one was near and there was no telling how long it had been this low. A strong athletic heart was a blessing, but even it has its limits. Spa's imperious words made the specter all the more ominous, and vigilance an absolute necessity.

Whispers could be heard in the ICU. "Well, he had a good life. Just keep him comfortable—let nature take its course." The sound of metal rollers, yanked on their tracks, signalled the staff closing white curtains promptly to keep the spectacle from view. A large black male nurse wheeled a rollaway bed out of the back door—a clean white

PART 1: MONTREAL, 1994

sheet over his cargo—leaving the cubicle across the way empty. I sat like a fixture, occasionally lifting my head to peer through the chink, and prayed that the same thing wouldn't happen to us. The nurse would normally have kicked me out, but familiarity seemed to have made me transparent. She seldom noticed me sitting mesmerized in the corner, or writing. The decision to move Bobby to Calgary took on an extra sense of urgency.

Moving a comatose patient demands significant support. The contract of the Federation of Med Residents of Quebec stipulated 30 days of service to be entitled to benefits, which Bobby did not have. Fearing the worst—he had fallen through the benefits crack as well—we went to the hospital social work office for help. It took little time to realize that the office was a PR trap—a disappointing waste of time.

3:00 P.M. NO SEIZURE ACTIVITY IN THE BRAIN, they said when the technologist completed the EEG. All systems were functioning as we waited for the surgical team to perform the tracheotomy, in ten minutes we were informed, and another EEG was scheduled for the morning.

Ten minutes turned into a two-hour wait. Finally, an anesthesiologist, respirologist and general surgery resident turned up through the back door of the ICU, and Bobby was whisked away to the amphitheatre. The operation was as quick as our cafeteria supper. Spa waited by the ICU door. "It went well," he said. "Bobby has a clear air passage; no trouble."

Infection following surgery was a serious concern, since Bobby had had a couple of bouts already following the departure of the friends who had held a wake for Bobby in Calgary. Bobby must be left alone until the morning EEG, I told Nan in the cafeteria. But Jen walked in and insisted on being there, on doing whatever she wished. It prompted an exchange on the common sense, or lack thereof, that had caused the poisoning in the first place. Agitated, she yelled, "I bear no responsibility for Bobby." She stormed out, blurting, "Tonight may be the last night."

The words struck us between our eyes. On more than one occasion,

MEDICAL MALADY

Bobby's BP dropped drastically. It could have gone unnoticed if we hadn't been around.

AS FAR BACK AS JULY 8, NAN HAD MADE A STRANGE OFFER to Gale: as an incentive for her to leave Montreal, Nan would pay our mortgage. Following the offer, a strange notation appeared in Bobby's chart, recorded by Pastor Perry, for the ICU doctors and nurses to read:

"Girlfriend's mother expressed concern to me over pt's father's state of mind…father does not believe that he is being told the truth concerning those events and appears to exhibit signs of paranoia … *Nan* suggested that…*father* may need some psychiatric support and perhaps evaluation (she is a psychiatrist)…"

Such activities—which I had interpreted as an effort to remove Gale from the scene and isolate me—prompted a closed-door meeting with Spa, our first. He invited his head nurse in. I said, "Jen's bizarre behavior suggests the anaphylaxic poisoning—the root cause of Bobby's hospitalization—doesn't seem accidental."

Predictably, Spa wasn't convinced. "If there is ever a court case, I would support Jen," he said, and advised me to see a psychiatrist before leaving Montreal.

"You mean Nan?" I asked, in sardonic seriousness.

"No, someone else," he belched. "One life ended, we have to save the other; this is a tragedy, but your kind have a good way of dealing with the dying and the dead."

The motive behind those words, and the goings-on that didn't involve Bobby's treatment—thus of least importance to us—were the subjects of long discussions between Gale and me. While Gale was more charitable, I had concluded that the remarks were intended either to provoke a reaction to prove Nan's point or to dehumanize victims to inflict further damage. We chose to let it go but waited anxiously for the moment to move Bobby.

If the ICU wasn't hell on earth, it certainly was a transition point to heaven. We were simply strangers in this domain. Nan, however, was at home in the scene and could use it to the fullest.

PART 1: MONTREAL, 1994

Spa announced that the earliest date for the move would be Friday, July 15. Why he relented to let us take Bobby back to Calgary remains a mystery. The questionable activities, however, left little doubt that Bobby would have passed through the transition point to heaven had he remained in that ICU another week. We couldn't wait a day longer.

8

ESCAPE

JULY 14. AN ESCAPE FROM MONTREAL WITH A COMATOSE son in tow wasn't assured, even for someone who'd managed complex projects for a living. Financing, lawyers, law enforcement, disposing of furniture, moving a car, terminating a lease—the to-do list was long. Project management took on a new meaning in the vortex of horror and hostility. Gale's presence kept me from being wrongfully committed to a psych ward, and helped in coordinating the multitude of activities in the brutality of time.

The benefits department of PCA, the integrated oil company I worked for, took an immediate interest, and after some investigation confirmed that Bobby, who was under twenty-five, could still be considered my dependent. Confederation Life Insurance Company would cover the cost of a hospital-to-hospital air-ambulance transfer.

STARS[3] ground ambulance would have a converted Learjet available. FHH's ICU transfer service confirmed that Bobby's transfer to Calgary was arranged, and a departure time was set for 2:30 P.M. the next day.

WHEN THE ANESTHESIA HAD WORN OFF following the tracheotomy, Bobby resumed semi-purposeful motions. Eyes wide open, hands and left leg bent, head slightly turned, he began to move his jaw—perhaps to communicate, perhaps to chew the ET tube that was no longer there—then fell deeper into sleep as night faded into morning.

PART 1: MONTREAL, 1994

We were at the ICU on time, but allowed in only after the doctors' rounds. Movements erratic, exhibiting gag reflexes, Bobby was more staring than looking. He became very active from time to time—indicating a wake cycle. The fever he had been having lately hadn't eased from 39°C. A cooling blanket was spread over him.

In late afternoon, Ratna waited patiently to help, while we waited inside for the results of the morning's EEG. Once outside the inner circle of the ICU, Dr. Crow had levelled with us. "What do you expect? Nan is trying to look after her daughter's interests." This time, Crow had both good news and bad. The good news: Bobby was seizure-free. The bad: It was unlikely he would improve much. His brain activity remained low, and his cortex could be damaged. There was a 95% chance he would spend the rest of his life in an institution. She seemed to want to prepare us for the worst.

A lawyer friend of Ratna's advised us on civil liability matters: jurisdiction, burden of proof, intent and negligence. However, knowing our interest rested in finding the truth that wasn't forthcoming, she was forthright. The justice system isn't designed to find the truth, she said, and she referred us to a criminal lawyer. His take was, "Going to the police is the only recourse; this merits an investigation and the police have the means." Testimony under oath would be a good start, a lie detector test even better, to determine what happened to Bobby on the night of Day Zero when Jen was the only other person in the apartment.

"We will be moving Bobby to Calgary," I said to the MNI's Dr. Antel, as he found us eating our last supper in the kosher cafeteria. "So throw at him the best Montreal has to offer in testing and treatment." Hands tied by hospital politics, he could provide nothing more than soothing words. Based on Scho's assessment, the prognosis was very bad, he said. He showed enormous empathy—a mark of a caring doctor who had taken the time to locate us. I pleaded. If he came up with a more aggressive treatment to control the seizures, would he let the doctors at the JGH and FHH know?

MEDICAL MALADY

FRIDAY, JULY 15. AN EARLY MORNING CALL FROM Sergeant Richard Robert of the Investigation branch of CUM (Communauté Urbaine de Montréal) police woke us. Following the advice of the criminal lawyer, I had gone to the police to determine what Nan and Dr. Spa were trying to protect Jen from, and the rationale for their symbiotic relationship. Constables Benoit and Masse were in the apartment within fifteen minutes. Neither was fluent in English, nor could we speak French. The communication gap couldn't be closed in forty minutes. Their next stops were the ICU, the Chinese restaurant, and Jen. Dr. Spa could stave them off in perfect French, pointing to Perry's note in the charts. It wasn't hard to imagine that the matter would end in futility, but the consolation was that we'd followed the lawyer's advice.

Arrangements to return Bobby's unpacked furniture to IKEA and to move the rest of his belongings back to Calgary kept us tied to the apartment all morning. Ratna brought her telephone books and two pairs of strong arms—Wishert's, her grad student's, and Vij's, her husband's. Bobby's apartment was abuzz.

We were about to leave when Gale received a phone call. Nan was on the other end, offering to return some of Bobby's valuables—gold-rim eyeglasses, his high school graduation ring and a gold chain—in exchange for four heavy bags from Bobby's apartment closet. We were puzzled; Jen had already collected her personal belongings nearly a week before. "What do the bags contain?" Gale wondered aloud.

"Camping gear," she was told. She agreed to deliver them to the ICU. Bobby would need his glasses when he came out of the coma.

Vij drove five human sardines in a tiny tin can—his Ford Escort—to the ICU, hauling the ransom. The bags were exchanged for the valuables left with the nurse.

Dr. Powell from STARS[4] had called already. The medical team was coordinated, and we could fly with Bobby. Dr. Crow received the same message. We breathed a sigh of relief. Crow gave me a handwritten letter on JGH letterhead—the release. Dr. Scho produced a handwritten letter as well, but Dr. Spa turned it back to get it typed, holding up the transfer. Scho said that the morning CAT scan results

PART 1: MONTREAL, 1994

had been normal. I asked if there was any hope. He was not optimistic. Chances were 99 out of 100 that Bobby would not recover, but in this case, he would be happy to be wrong. He said that he'd consulted with Dr. Antel, and had gone over all Bobby's treatment. He'd asked his colleague if they could have done anything differently. The answer he said he'd received was no. I asked him to keep Bobby in mind, and that if he had any new thoughts, to communicate them to FHH and to me. I gave him my address and telephone number. He wrote his on the back of a blood gas requisition.

2:10 P.M. THE STARS MEDICAL TEAM—three members in blue Nomex coveralls who had flown into Dorval—was driven to the hospital in an ambulance. We remained by the ICU, awaiting instructions while the team was briefed on the patient's condition, medicine regimen and paperwork. It took time to get organized—to be certain they wouldn't run short of medicine, oxygen and or supplies during the long flight back to Calgary. With the patient transfer protocol completed, the ICU gave up control, and STARS took over. The ICU nurse stayed with Bobby until they wheeled him into the waiting yellow box of an ambulance, bearing the insignia of a smug white snake around a white staff at a blue crossroad.

Ratna, Gale and I rushed into a waiting blue taxi, in fast pursuit of the box that kept vanishing in thick Metropolitan Boulevard traffic. The ambulance chose not to use the flashers, though it moved just as fast in a city of speedsters. Our cabby followed it to the Shell Aero Centre, right up to the blue-and-white striped Learjet parked on the tarmac.

Embarking into the air ambulance presented a challenge for the team. There was no turnaround room for the rollaway stretcher. Bobby's head needed to be at the bow, facing the medics, requiring a breech entry—feet first. The pilot and the co-pilot joined in to help position the immobilized passenger. A rhythmic motion of the nurse's right hand squeezing the oxygen bag lifted his chest, barely visible through the blankets and the straps. Her left hand held the med-satchel high in the air, allowing gravity to infuse the life-saving fluids.

Her eyes never lost their focus on life, and vitals, as we stood steps away, speechless, motionless, at one with Bobby. Ratna organized our luggage to be carried into the plane.

Bobby was on the stretcher, and the accompanying appurtenances that kept him alive settled in, when the signal came for us to board. One step up and we found ourselves in the gill of the crammed twin-engine plane. The stretcher and the tangled equipment took nearly all the available space in its belly, with the exception of the nurse's seat near his head, and a bench at the stern past his feet. There was just enough room to crouch and squeeze past. We were asked to take the corners. The reason quickly became clear.

Dr. Shepard, jammed between Gale and me, turned to the cargo hold behind the bench to check the oxygen supply and other unrecognizable equipment. Direct access to the patient secured, he held the rotameter in his hand, an instrument that indicated O_2 flow to the ventilator. The paramedic did a final calibration check.

4:08 P.M. The plane took off just as soon as the team was in perfect coordination. Paralyzed with Norcuron, Bobby seemed stable. His open eyes were now taped shut. It was important to do this as the eyes dry out if they are kept open without blinking and can be damaged permanently. The flight physician soon determined that the patient needed bagging; the small ventilator seemed unreliable. Bobby's heartbeat was fine, but his BP and temperature were unknown.

An hour into the flight, Bobby had consumed one tiny cylinder of the oxygen that maintained his O_2 saturation at 95%. Almost two hours into the flight, his vitals were stable. He lay motionless as the epitomes of professionalism on his right—the doctor, the paramedic and the nurse—kept a close watch on the five drip lines and watched the ventilator, now working again. The tiny machine emulated human breathing—inflating his lungs faster than normal with a jerk, relaxing momentarily, then exhaling somewhat normally. The second O_2 cylinder got low, and the equilibrium was disrupted in a flurry of activity.

Moving a comatose patient by air ambulance is not without risk. Bobby could expire on the flight. However, the farther we got from

PART 1: MONTREAL, 1994

Montreal the more hopeful we felt. And when there is hope, there is life. Keeping Bobby in Montreal was no longer an option. We were caught between the ogre and the women, in the transition point to heaven, convinced that Bobby wouldn't be with us had we left him there. That became apparent on more occasions than one. Our only option was to transfer him to Calgary and give his treatment a fresh start—in a familiar teaching hospital, with a known set of home-city doctors—with family and friends nearby.

A strong headwind stretched the trip to the limit. An hour from arrival, Bobby was on the last of the four bottles of O_2 on board. How long would it last? The question remained unanswered. He was back on the ventilator—his chest rising much faster than it was coming down. An occasional scurry of activity would spike our attention; the rescue team wasn't sure whether the O_2 was going in.

"Forty minutes to landing," the pilot announced. A severe thunderstorm loomed in Calgary. The headwind grew stronger, turning the three-and-a-half hour journey into a four-and-a-half hour one. Bobby had been lying in the same stretched position throughout. The ventilator finally gave up the ghost, leaving his life in the hands of the nurse—alternating much more frequently now as she squeezed the O_2 bag. With the Norcuron running low, Bobby started to move, adding further challenges to the work of the medical team.

6:30 P.M. IN THE EYE OF A SEVERE THUNDERSTORM, the Learjet landed. With a nerve-shattering touchdown, it sped along the runway on reverse thrust, repelling droplets that sparkled by the millions on the tiny windows, refracting landing lights. The plane taxied directly into the Shell Aero Centre hangar. A thunderous crackle crossing the bituminous sky welcomed Bobby home.

An ambulance whisked his stretcher away the minute it disembarked and transferred. A bed and a nursing team were waiting for him in the FHH ICU. We stayed behind for the luggage in tumultuous rain, and then hired a cab to follow the uncertain road in a darkness that shrouded the summer sun.

PART 2:
CALGARY, 1994

9

DREAM

CALGARY SEEMED LIKE A DREAM—a fresh medical team, newer equipment and facilities, just the picture we'd painted in our minds. I couldn't help but feel that Bobby's chances of recovery would be better—a lot better. Quebec had come to symbolize certain death; Alberta offered hope, life.

A cordial hospital admissions staffer greeted me with paperwork that evaporated time. Gale, as anxious as I was, left me at the admitting office and went looking for the ICU waiting room, dragging our luggage behind her. She ran into friends who had brought the rest of our besieged family—Nihar, Mon and Neilly—in their minivan. She was relieved to see them—as I was when I joined them on the ICU floor after all the paperwork.

The protocol here was similar to that in Montreal—a waiting room and an access telephone at a distance from an unimposing entrance. Two people were allowed into the ICU at a time. Gale and I went in to find a relaxed atmosphere. They weren't busy, and almost everyone knew Bobby. Attending nurse Maggie had worked with him in his final year of med school; the young resident Wendy was a year ahead of the Peccaries—so named for the mascot that symbolized Bobby's graduating class of 1994. Bobby looked peaceful despite the arduous flight, deeper in sleep, or perhaps they had pushed a mega-dose of neuromuscular Norcuron—Pavulon they called it here. STARS, they told us, had delivered Bobby in a hemodynamically stable condition. His condition hadn't deteriorated in transit.

PART 2: CALGARY, 1994

The rest of the family was allowed in for a short period. "Everything will be all right," Nihar assured, stroking Bobby's comatose forehead. Neilly and Mon stood frozen a few steps away. Gale took them back out to join the friends, who took them all home. I decided to stay. Another family friend, having some treatment at the hospital, offered me a ride later.

A casual conversation with Wendy brought a staggering revelation. Bobby, she said, had had a cardiorespiratory arrest (CRA)—in the JGH ER—lasting five to seven minutes. I'd heard no such thing in Montreal. Bobby never had a heart attack, I protested in shock, struggling to take in the news. My understanding, I said, was that the ER had been unable to find his pulse for less than 30 seconds, prompting a few precautionary chest compressions.

"Were you there?" she countered.

"No," I said, "but I've spoken to two of the three ER doctors who were."

"Sure." Her tone was dismissive.

The spectre of Spa appeared in my mind. "I will talk to Dr. Sand in the morning." Did he tell him what he had told me? That patients like Bobby seize, seize, seize and die? Or that his life ended; you can do whatever with his body? After all, a wake had been held for him already!

Those loaded words weren't exactly examples of the kind of professionalism I was accustomed to in the paradigm of my workplace. Would he repeat them to Sand, or simply send him the charts to back up whatever he'd said? I didn't know. I needed to sort it all out rationally, logically.

A cardiac arrest meant that there had been no flow of blood to Bobby's brain, no oxygen—anoxia. For a brain to remain oxygen-starved for five to seven minutes would be a dead serious matter. The ER doctors had told me that Bobby had suffered a respiratory arrest, that is, only a partial loss of oxygen—hypoxia. Wendy couldn't have fabricated it—why would she? She had been told either directly or indirectly.

If Wendy's version were true, Bobby would not have squeezed my hand in Montreal on request—he would likely be brain dead. The release papers made no mention of cardiac arrest. Dr. Spa did not author, or sign, the Montreal discharge papers; he had written precious little in the charts, although he was responsible for nearly all critical decisions made in the Montreal ICU, and had gotten directly involved every step of the way. He had had Scho and Crow write the discharge papers, though he spoke to Sand himself.

The JGH ER and ICU charts were nowhere in sight. Wendy and Maggie appeared guarded about the issue. They were depending on clinical evaluation, short on experience and long on hearsay, having dismissed an important link to patient history—parents. In Stampede City—in a transient province of cowboys and drilling rigs—fathers were often stereotyped as hedonistic, wallet-centred morons, preoccupied with hockey, beer and sex. The closed communication in a closed system became stifling.

I headed home late in the night, pondering. Imposing a drug-induced condition on unsuspecting patients wasn't unheard of in Montreal in the '50s. Had the JGH ICU done it in good faith, or was it done to facilitate a fast transition? When that failed, had Spa lied to Sand and passed on the false clinical history?

10

NIGHTMARE

SATURDAY, JULY 16. "QUITE A BIT OF 'MOVEMENT' LAST NIGHT," the ICU nurse told us when she greeted us in the morning. The descriptor was unfamiliar to me. Was this movement seizures, I wondered, or myoclonus? They'd given Bobby Pavulon, but maintained anticonvulsants at the therapeutic level. Bobby's temperature had shot up on the flight, but descended upon arrival—perhaps it had been the cooling effect of the high altitude. Two different antibiotics, an alcohol bath, and glycol cooling blankets—over his legs and underneath him—maintained his temperature near normal. It was a good sign. Mon had come with me to the hospital, and she and I hoped that Bobby would come out of this spell on his own soon. She would start med school this fall; the morning physiotherapist was her biochemistry classmate at the University of Calgary.

I hoped the resident—anemic residency training for a fellow Peccary in crisis—would call in the staff neurologist. Almost every neurologist in this small community of neurologists knew Bobby, and through his association, we knew of them. Dr. Lee, whose son was a Peccary, was the neurologist on call. I hoped he'd treat Bobby as "one of their own," and carry out the necessary diagnostic testing.

Lee examined Bobby late in the morning. Nerves deadened by the neuromuscular blocker failed to respond to painful stimuli. Lee scribbled his observations in the chart: "Curiously, he does not move at all in response to painful stimulation."—and delivered a devastating diagnosis: decorticate. No cerebral cortex activity, nothing that makes one human. That handwritten bombshell might as well have been written in blood when I saw it much later. I felt the shock—an act of betrayal.

When the Pavulon wore off, Lee nowhere in sight, Bobby displayed his typical sleep–wake cycle, just as he had in Montreal. In wake cycle, he would become restless, and respond to my voice and touch. I'd ask him to relax, and he would, several times. Nurses diligently noted these moments in his chart. I wondered if the doctors had actually read the chart each time they went into the room. Agitation was an indication of Bobby's discomfort, for instance, when the ventilator wasn't working properly, and there wasn't enough oxygen. Nurses were free with Valium, whatever the cause. It kept things under control—for patient and nurses alike—no need to scurry. Protective elbow-pads abated damage from the movements. Bobby was clean-shaven, much thinner, much more adjusted to the trachea tube. His stomach was kept in suction. The nurse gave me a shopping list—Walkman, socks, shaving cream, deodorant, toothbrush and toothpaste. Moments vanished as we were chased out between shifts, or asked to leave when they worked on him. We looked for doctors and decision makers, and fielded questions from family, friends and curiosity seekers. No kosher cafeteria here, no Sabbath elevator. FHH was secular.

JULY 17. BOBBY SEEMED RECOVERED FROM THE AIR-AMBULANCE trip. When in wake cycle, he opened his eyes and moved them from side to side in what appeared to be attempts to grasp the conversations going on around him. He hated the cooling blankets. He pulled out the pipe—much to the annoyance of the nurse—and blue glycol-water flowed over the bleach-white sheet. She pushed Valium. He couldn't cry, although at times I'd see a teardrop or two roll down from the corner of his eyes. He couldn't scream, or tell her what was bothering him; he could only show signs of distress through agitation.

Evening brought a tornado of change. The nurse took Bobby off the ventilator and put him on a trachea-cradle. Within minutes, his O_2 saturation dropped to 80%; he was like a fish out of water.

PART 2: CALGARY, 1994

He became so bronchospastic—couldn't breathe on his own—that a respirologist had to be called in to bag. Nurses weren't free with information, nor with access to the ICU. Bobby's eyes grew larger and moved from side to side as they lowered the Dilantin as well—the all-important anticonvulsant.

Beyond agitation by late evening, Bobby became combative. Was he trying to tell us something through his actions, actions I had never seen before? The nurses used straps to restrain his hands, to keep him from pulling out his trachea tube. His legs were free, and he wedged them between the mattress and the rails. His eyes were active, not focused on anything in particular. His temperature and heart rate shot way up.

"He could hurt himself," I blurted out. Had he been trying to wake up? Had he been in dire distress? My questioning led to the discovery of drip lines that had run dry. Medications weren't going in. The nurse noticed that too. She pushed Valium and recorded her observations in his chart: "Strong response to painful stimuli, tended to settle when stroked his hair, seemed to be aware as he repositioned himself."

JULY 18. AN AIR OF DOOM GREETED US. The nurse noted "tremors," and Bobby wasn't responding as he had the day before. We were summoned to a family meeting at noon following the rounds. No such meetings had ever been held for us in Montreal.

We walked into a roomful of people around a table: Sand—the ICU chief; Susan—the ICU nurse; Marge—the patient care manager; Scott—the first-year neurology resident; Drs. Doi and Lee. The bearded, barrel-chested chief was a middle-age doctor with steely eyes and a vise grip over the group. He delivered the message, recorded verbatim in the chart, as the others nodded in agreement.

"I have reviewed Bobby's chart with Dr. Spa [by telephone], Drs. Doi and Lee. We all agree that Bobby has no cortex function, there has been no movement, the chance for recovery to a meaningful functional state is nil. We will take Bobby off the ventilator and move him to the neurology ward within the next few days. Once discharged from the ICU, he will not be re-admitted."

Gale keeled over to cover her ears as the barrel fired on. "Bobby will be taken off antibiotics. If his heart stops, he will not be revived. If his lungs get infected, he will not be treated."

He paused, as if to drive home the fact that Bobby would be left to die. That gave me an opening: "Bobby was never anoxic, he was hypoxic. He never had a heart attack. There is a huge difference in prognosis. Don't pull the plug on Bobby."

"We will continue to provide the best possible care, as we do for all patients."

"Bobby was a medical student here; surely he should get some consideration."

The team marched out, following their leader. Gale began to cry. I yelled, "If there is a one in a million chance, give him that chance."

Sand noted my desperate plea for help in the chart, yet refused to provide further neurological assessment.

I approached our family physician, and Bobby's neurology preceptor at the Health Sciences Centre. They referred me to the chairman of neurology, to no avail. A neuro-consult in the ICU was by invitation only, and the invitation had to come from the ICU chief. We were losing precious time.

We dragged ourselves back into the ICU. Bobby's seizures were worse—arching back, twitching, shaking, thrashing. I requested another meeting with the medical team. We had nothing to lose by trying a different handle. Gupta was back from Boston. I asked him to be present with his wife, a psychologist, with the hope of securing an alternative medical opinion.

6:00 P.M. THE VENTILATOR SEEMED ATTACHED and functioning when I returned to the ICU with Mon; Gale had stayed home. She had lost faith in a system that allowed such cruelty to go on without proper diagnosis and treatment. Bobby looked limp; perhaps he'd had a Valium push. Yet his eyes, lips, left foot and hand were all twitching. Since Montreal had raised the dose of Dilantin to the therapeutic level—it was noted in his chart that Bobby was a high metabolizer of the drug—the twitching had stopped.

PART 2: CALGARY, 1994

I had support in the evening meeting: Dr. Smith—Dean of the Faculty of Medicine—Mon, Gupta and his wife. Sand, however, was unshakable. He simply repeated the morning's decree in a milder tone. Gupta requested the intervention of Dr. Mukherjee, an independent neurologist in the city whom he knew. He was an outsider and not a part of the team. Sand reluctantly agreed.

Concerned that the seizures were exacerbating the damage to Bobby's brain before the independent neurologist had a chance to consult, I asked them to reinstate anticonvulsants to the therapeutic level. They nearly fell over each other to storm out. It's inhuman to let Bobby seize, I cried out. Dean Smith remained to hear my grievance and a *Calgary Herald* reporter walked in. Gupta had invited him before leaving home.

The nurse had noted in the chart that Bobby had attempted to sit up while she gave him a bed-bath—". . .his eyes opened wider when his name was called." She had brought her observations to Dr. Doi's attention, but the movements were dismissed as "non-purposeful." The nurse's notes and observations were ignored, while the monstrosity of misinformation marched on to the drumbeat of a self-fulfilling prophecy.

11

STATUS EPILEPTICUS

JULY 19. ANXIOUS HOURS PASSED AS WE AWAITED the independent neurologist. Meanwhile, the *Calgary Herald* published our plea, verbatim, to hold off the withdrawal of life support. "All we want is for the hospital to maintain the steady state that he is in for may be one, two, three months to give him a chance to recover . . . and we [the family] would like to start a prayer service for him in all denominations across the city until he comes around."

The city responded from all corners, and the hospital relented, a bit. Although we weren't told, an EEG was done on July 18. Dr. M. Lee—Lee's sister—reported, and we discovered much later, that "the EEG also shows some reactivity to painful stimulation, which is a relatively good prognostic sign." Her words essentially refuted her brother's diagnosis of "decorticate." Sand wrote in the chart—"NR [nonresponsive] to pain x4 [in all four limbs]"—ignoring the nurse's notes, which read, "withdrawal of all four limbs to painful stimuli; pt's [patient's] eyes open wider c [with] calling."

The medical team met for an update following rounds early in the afternoon—Sand, Doi, Zia, Sagan, Sandra, and the ICU nurse were present, but no neurologist. The chief repeated the grim pronouncement: . . . outlook very poor; Bobby would be taken off the ventilator and put on a trachea cradle with oxygen; he would have to breathe by himself—there would be no return to life support.

Through his nurse, Sand handed me an article written by Dr. E. Wijdicks[5], a U.S. researcher. It suggested withdrawal of life support

PART 2: CALGARY, 1994

for patients exhibiting myoclonus status (non-stop myoclonus from anoxia), claiming that all forty patients who exhibited it—following out-of-hospital cardiac arrest—had died.

But Bobby had never had a heart attack, much less an out-of-hospital one. Buried deep in the documents—and revealed later to us—was that Sand had all but acknowledged to the nurses that Bobby was having status epilepticus (non-stop seizures from hypoxia; patients do not die but suffer brain injury if they remain untreated) and not myoclonus status. The gulf of difference between Wijdicks's patients and Bobby brushed aside, the ICU was about to become the Serengeti of the civilized world—where bringing down one served many. Wijdicks's article seemed to be the ammunition poised to extinguish our hope and Bobby's life.

I begged them to keep Bobby on the ventilator until Dr. Mukherjee had a chance to examine him. The hospital ignored me and put him on the trachea cradle with 50% oxygen, claiming that they were acting in the patient's interest. Bobby coughed, gagged, vomited and wheezed. His heart rate rocketed, blood oxygen dropped, and streaks of bowel movements, and blood in his urine, appeared from the strain. To make matters worse, the seizures didn't cease—they intensified. He experienced rapid eyelid blinking, chewing motions in the mouth, agitation, arching back, legs over the rails; he was wheezing and coughing out thick, blood-tinged sputum.

DIRECTIONLESS, I DROVE to my office on the 27th floor of P-C Centre in the heart of downtown Calgary. Nearly three weeks of absence had created a mountain of mail. Going hastily through it, I came across the name Adolfo, a colleague of mine in the West Tower who had lost one of his sons—about the same age as Bobby—the year before. They had given the young man a 2% chance for survival before pulling the plug. For Bobby, the chance was nil. Adolfo had accepted his fate. He asked me to get hold of Russ Kelly, the EAP[6] counselor who had helped him get through the ordeal.

My appointment with Russ the next day was on the 20th floor of the Centre. A straight shooter with penetrating eyes, he narrated his life's trepidations to break the ice, and paused to listen to Bobby's. Knowing that the hospital had given Adolfo's son better odds before turning off the life support, he asked, "What are you doing here?"

"I am trying to . . . I don't think I am winning this one."

"What if he slips away?"

I couldn't respond.

"If he does, you may regret not being there for the rest of your life."

"I know," I mumbled.

Russ was single, in his fifties. He knew the value of life with a son, and turned up the pressure. "If I were you," he continued, "I would be with my son as much as possible. If you choose not to be there, that's different."

He knew that if I were at Bobby's bedside, I could continue to fight on. I rushed to my office. Cheryl—our secretary whose son, an only child, had been injured in an unfortunate accident—hurried in for an update. "I am leaving," I said to her. "I won't be coming back for the next couple of days." She didn't respond. Her eyes filled with tears, and she gave me an abrupt hug before I could step out.

ARMS RESTRAINED IN A CARDIAC CHAIR like a subdued prisoner, Bobby appeared wilted. They had lowered his oxygen in the trachea cradle to 25%. He was warm to the touch, perspiring, coughing and wheezing. His breathing was shallow but rapid. Moments later, the sedation wore off and the tremors took over—shaking, quivering and agitating. The incessant thrashing blistered his heels as his high-pitched wheezing and coughing reverberated off the walls, projecting past the doors into the open hallway.

The nurse announced that a young woman was waiting outside. Gale and I opened the ICU door and the young woman embraced us. In one breath, she said her name was Liz, and that she'd come as soon as she could after reading the article about Bobby in the morning newspaper. She too was anaphylactic to peanuts; she had nearly died

PART 2: CALGARY, 1994

from a kiss of death from her husband. Liz, a concerned Calgarian, came to offer support, for which we were grateful.

BOBBY'S INCESSANT SEIZING PROMPTED me to ask the nurse to check the blood Dilantin levels. No analyses had been done, not since July 15. Yet without checking the levels, the ICU had no basis to mercilessly lower anticonvulsants—900 mg on July 17, 600 mg on July 18, 300 mg on July 19 and 20—before turning them off altogether and watching him seize, seize, seize . . . and die.

Bobby endured yet another day of the dreaded status epilepticus without being assessed by a neurologist. Mukherjee asked for more "data"—presumably the Montreal ER report that wasn't made available. Desperate, I asked the nurse to call in the staff neurologist, the one who'd explained to me over the telephone the previous day that "Myoclonus and seizures are two intersecting circles; seizures originate from and affect critical parts of the brain, whereas myoclonus originates from and affects the brain stem; myoclonus couldn't hurt much but seizures is another matter." Sand answered the nurse's page from the comfort of his home, but steadfastly refused to help. We wondered if Bobby would survive another night.

12

STONE HEAD

"BOBBY WILL COME THROUGH." Dr. Samuel Weiss poured his words of optimism into our ears in the family waiting room. "The human brain is very resilient; it can relearn everything," he said. Sam knew what he was talking about; he was a brain researcher who worked in the Health Sciences laboratories, next door to Dr. Wolfram Tetzlaff, whom Bobby had worked for during his pre-med and med years in Calgary. Slicing rat brain and spinal cord and preparing slides for researchers to study cell regeneration were of enormous interest to Bobby. This work had led to his residency position in neurology at the MNI. When Sam heard about Bobby's condition, he couldn't stay away, and we were grateful for his visit.

While his words were reassuring to our ears, the old clinicians weren't buying them. Clinicians often dismiss researchers, whose knowledge is based on mouse models, not humans. They continue to work with their antiquated knowledge base, too proud to seek new information from their junior colleagues, or so it seemed.

Wolf, Bobby's old supervisor, called from Ottawa. He shared Sam's optimism: "There is some hope. The brain stem center overrides the cortex sometimes; shakes go away. Good chance Bobby is intellectually intact. The brain typically functions at 80–100% O_2 saturation; 30–60% is enough for survival. At 25%, however, the brain stops function, yet survives; but below 12% it dies." Bobby's saturation had never been below 30% and his heart stopped for less than 30 seconds—Koh had confirmed that in Montreal.

PART 2: CALGARY, 1994

THE INDEPENDENT NEUROLOGIST, whom we had never met, assessed Bobby at long last. Sam came to the meeting room where the medical team assembled: Drs. Doi, Scott, the head nurse, the attending nurse and Mukherjee. Sand was conspicuously absent. Frail and near retirement, the neurologist gave his briefing in a vacuum of clinical history: "Bobby had had a triple-barrelled gun shot at him during his anaphylactic attack: his heart did not pump enough blood, his lungs stopped and his blood vessels constricted."

The briefing was long on generalities and short on specifics. It was obvious to me that Mukherjee, who didn't appear to be condescending or dismissive, had not received the "data" he had requested.

"We need to take one day at a time," he continued. The myoclonic jerks could stop in 10 days, but he was not optimistic. His prognosis: Bobby was heading toward a persistent vegetative state—PVS[7]. As devastating as it was for me to hear his prognosis, I had reason to believe that he had been thorough enough to read the nurses' notes here in Calgary, and that he'd slow the ICU's haste. With a diagnosis of PVS, he said, international code calls for a 30-day wait before life support could be withdrawn. They had to give Bobby ten more days before reducing him to a collection of organs, ripe for harvest, I thought. The second opinion let the rightful owner of the organs maintain possession, giving him a temporary lease on life.

Mukherjee prescribed a new medication, Clonazepam—an antimyoclonic seizure drug—dosage of which he had to keep low and build up slowly because he had no control of Bobby's airway. They had taken him off the ventilator. The tablets needed crushing and feeding through the NG tube, but his stomach wasn't functioning. Whatever was being fed was passing right through—the seizures made him incontinent. It would take a while to build up the drug to the therapeutic level. Meanwhile, the electric storm raged on in his brain.

That night, I enquired about Dilantin. The attending nurse informed me that both Dilantin and Phenobarbital had been completely discontinued, removing any defense against seizures—and seizures indeed begat more seizures. Bobby was consumed in constant tremors. His eyes quivered, the chewing movements persisted in his mouth, his foot curled downward in jerking motion, he arched back with agitation. Wheezing and coughing incessantly, his respiration soared to 36 breaths per minutes, his heart rate raced to 148. They lowered his oxygen. Bobby was running a non-stop marathon in bed. Pushed to the limit, he developed tachycardia[8].

JULY 21. NO VENTILATOR ASSIST. Catheter removed. Nurse was unable to sedate him anymore. It is a miracle Bobby survived the night. We were called in to yet another one-way meeting with the medical team.

"We will be moving Bobby to the ward tonight," Sand informed us.

"For Bobby to move to the ward, his gut must work, so the Clonazepam has a chance to . . .".

"Since you like to be in control, our proposal is for you to take Bobby home."

"How do we take him home? We are not medical people," Gale and I piped in, in unison. "Can you tell me whether a coma patient belongs in the hospital or at home?"

Suddenly Marge found her voice, "You can take him to Care West . . ."

I pleaded for anticonvulsants and an EEG instead. Sand marched out in disbelief at our audacious challenge to the superior power—others followed. Bobby's respiration and heart rate climbed further. He began to pant, and the nurse found it hard to keep the drip lines going.

Calls from reporters for the story and offers of expertise from concerned citizens came pouring in, but what we needed was an ethics advocate at arm's length from the hospital. Health Sciences had an ethics department, but the committee members—Michael and Ellen—were on vacation. Sam and Alice—the parents of Mon's classmate—suggested that we transcend the mortals and plead directly to the ultimate Christian authority. We joined them in prayer through the night in the ICU family room.

PART 2: CALGARY, 1994

Our prayers were answered in part the next day. Bobby had longer gaps between seizure spells. Sand wasn't around, and Doi decided against sending him to the ward when he developed arrhythmia. One more night of one-on-one care in the ICU and a gradual increase in the dose of Clonazepam produced longer sleep cycles during the lulls, and as he slept, he had breaks from the seizure spells. His vitals were better in the morning. Rest had done some good.

Unfortunately, the sleep cycle wore off in the morning and the seizures overtook with a vengeance. Bobby was flailing away as they removed all monitors—O_2 sat, heart and BP—in preparation for transfer to the ward. No vitals, no alarm, no hope. He was perspiring in profusion, his body temperature felt high to touch, and his heart rate was higher. He was incontinent. Bobby's marathon race could end at any time with heart failure.

In utter frustration and desperation, I asked Wendy why they hadn't tried to control Bobby's temperature.

"His brain's temperature-control mechanism is shot."

Kicked out of the ICU for rounds, we huddled in the waiting room.

"The doctors can do whatever they want: you are not Bobby's legal guardian," a visitor we didn't know piped into our conversation of despair.

Mystified, I replied, "Bobby is still our dependent. We are his parents, paying all the bills."

"Don't matter a hoot," he suggested. "See Legge and Chisholm, lawyers."

I noted the name, but I was not about to leave in search of a lawyer. The fight boiled down to a half a milligram of Clonazepam tablet at a time.

The last charade of a family conference took place in unit 103, with a pronouncement from Sand. "Bobby will be moved to the ward this afternoon, no ifs ands or buts."

"Sending a coma patient to the ward is a death sentence," I pleaded. "Bobby isn't stable, he cannot call for help in distress; he cannot press a button; he is asthmatic."

Their silence prompted me to carry on: "What do you think is the definition of coma? Is Bobby in a coma?"

"Yes. Bobby is in a coma."

"Well then, does he belong in a ward, or in the ICU?"

The hospital social worker, Sandra, and the nurse, Laura, remained mute; their presence added no value. I addressed the walls: "I will be meeting with Dr. Kinsella to check if a coma patient belongs to the unit or in the ICU."

They headed for the door in a rush, just as I mentioned Kinsella. Marg was more concerned about the media. She wrote her home telephone number in the charts and instructed the nurses to call her if the media made contact, or if we tried to bring the media into the unit.

I had called Kinsella, director of bioethics, in the morning; he was on his way to a meeting. Unable to see us, he answered my questions over the telephone and agreed to meet us in the afternoon.

"Do you think a coma patient belongs in a ward, or does he belong in the ICU?"

"A coma patient does not belong in a ward; he should be in the ICU."

"What happens if someone runs a marathon for a week?"

"He dies in exhaustion."

"That is what's been happening to Bobby. They are trying to exhaust him to death!"

Gale and I met Kinsella—a tall, white-haired man over sixty—in the afternoon. He had obviously had conversations with Sand by then: "Dr. Sand was a very good student of mine; I have every confidence in him . . ."

Our conversation, terminated prematurely, led me to the conclusion that medical ethics within an arm's length of the hospital is a myth, embraced in a system accustomed to stroking itself in the comfort of elegant offices. Lesson learned, Gale and I headed for the gallows of grief.

13

REBIRTH

NEUROLOGY WARD, JULY 22, 3 P.M. They wheeled Bobby's bed to a semi-private room. Within an hour, the staff realized that his thrashing, wheezing, seizing, and panting, and the raspy whistling sounds emanating from the trachea tube were causing undue stress to the patient in the next bed. They moved him to a private room. No extra charge; it was the hospital's decision.

Dr. Zac, the staff neurologist, Dr. Bern, the neurology resident, and the ward's head nurse, Marg, met us in the small consulting room farthest from the exit. I heard Marg say that there were eight patients to a nurse—three registered nurses (RNs) in a ward of 33 patients. The rest of her words were a buzz, drowned out by the shout of a female patient summoning the nurse every minute like clockwork. A slouched old man in the hallway attempted to maneuver his wheelchair aimlessly with one hand; the other appeared flaccid and futile.

Our nonresponsive patient was vastly different from others afflicted with strokes, aneurysms or similar brain injuries that made the unit morbidly depressing. Bobby simply didn't stand a chance of getting attention; besides, young patients like him were few and far between. He would wake up, I was sure, but until he did, we wouldn't know the multiplicity of injuries that the "non-intervention" had inflicted upon him, together with those he had suffered in Montreal. The ICU nurses were knowledgeable in all aspects of the patient care that had kept him alive to this day. The ward nurse, on the other hand, couldn't administer a Ventolin bronchodilator through his trachea tube. She hadn't done it for a patient like him before. In fact, she'd never seen a patient like Bobby in the neuro ward.

He continued to flail away, sweating profusely. The NG tube taped to his nose shook like a misaligned steering wheel, with no monitors of any kind to gauge his vitals. The nurse would manually take them when she had a chance—every hour, we hoped.

Marg was stern and self-righteous. "Nature will take care of him," she declared, within earshot of Gale, "and ease the passage. All his treatment is for treating them," she said, as she glanced from the corner of her eyes, perhaps to get a reaction from Gale, and went on. "He is getting enough treatment."

THE NEXT MORNING, BOBBY WASN'T IN HIS ROOM. I hurried to the nurse's station. Rudely, a passing nurse asked me to wait, leaving me wondering the worst. *God, have they eased the passage already, or have they taken him to the morgue for his convenience?* Minutes seemed like millennia. I yelled, "Could someone tell me where my son is?"

"He is taking a tub bath," a drawly female voice yelled back from behind the shoulder-high circular counter.

I returned to his room and resumed pacing back and forth between the windowpanes overlooking the parking lot and the hallway. A door creaked open across the hall. And there he was, lying on his back in a sac, knees tucked in close to the chest like a lobster in a trap, hoisted from the tub with a winch, all towel-dried and powdered. Smiling, the nurse started pushing the jig toward me. Our Christmas present was being delivered all over again, nearly twenty-three years later, by a mechanical stork.

"Thank God, he is alive." I closed my eyes, inviting the past.

TURKEY DINNER had been served in Gale's room in the maternity ward at the Sarnia General Hospital on December 24, 1971, the day after Bobby was born. I was allowed to bring my food tray from the cafeteria. Following our meal, they brought the baby in Santa's large furry red sock with a wide white trim. Small white plastic cubes with

PART 2: CALGARY, 1994

rounded corners encircled his neck. The sides of the beads spelled out his full name, in red and blue letters. "Merry Christmas, Gale. Here's a present for you," they said.

Wouldn't it be fitting, I wished, if he were to wake up now and celebrate a second birth? The wish remained buried, deep in the canyon of coma.

Powdered Clonazepam tablets were administered through the NG tube and Ventolin through the trachea, shortly after he was repatriated to his bed. Physiotherapy and doctors' visits followed. Bobby remained quiet at first, but then the demons of seizures and restlessness started up all over again.

In the days following, his seizures became more myoclonic, appearing in spurts rather than in a continuous tremor. They increased the dosage of Clonazepam from half a milligram to one, which began to show results. His shakes changed, appearing on both sides of his body, and his head and shoulders exhibited unusual movements that hadn't been there before—*ataxia* they called it. Regardless, he remained non-responsive and comatose.

SUNDAY, JULY 24. Bath and medications were over with when I arrived at nine in the morning. Bobby was in a reclined position on an orange vinyl chair, for the first time since moving to the ward. His eyes were closed, left leg folded, hands pinned to his side by the rails that held him in place. A new white surgical tape on the tip of his nose held in the NG tube. The trachea tube made a slight whistling sound, not like the foundry bellows that had run full tilt in the ICU. Dozing but looking brighter, Bobby showed no signs of seizure. He seemed to be in a sleep cycle. I tiptoed in, set my Hilroy logbook on the window ledge, and slouched on the chair against the wall at the foot of his bed, careful not to interrupt the calm, yet desperately wanting him to come out of the spell.

An hour later, a pleasantly plump lady in white garb walked in and addressed him as if she'd known him for years. "How are you doing, Bobby?"

He seemed to be expecting her. He smiled. His big brown eyes partially opened.

She must be a physiotherapist, I thought. I asked her name.

"Marian," she said, without paying much attention to me.

I'd never seen her before, and no physiotherapist was scheduled on a Sunday.

He connected with her instantly as she lowered the side rails.

"Can you move your left leg, Bobby?"

He straightened out his leg consciously. I sat up to pay closer attention to the goings-on.

She exercised his leg, up to his chest and down a few times.

"Now, can you move your right leg?"

He folded his right leg, and she repeated the exercise.

The same routine went on with his arms. She helped him move his hand over his head and down to his chest a few times.

"Okay, you're done for the day; see ya, Bobby." She was at the door about to leave when I jumped out of my stupor and rushed to whisper in her ear.

"Hey, he has obeyed your verbal command!"

"Oh, that's all reflex." She walked out softly, the way she'd come in.

No sooner had I returned to my chair, pondering if Marian's visit had been a dream, than a monsoon of realities rushed in. The entire neurology ward seemed to descend on the floor of room #1019. Could Marian have visited the nurse's station that fast? First came the nurses. Close behind were the resident and the staff neurologist. Others peered through the door.

The nurses: "Can you squeeze my hand, Bobby?" A hard squeeze followed.

"Bobby, can you lift your right leg?" He raised his right leg.

"Can you lift your left arm?" He raised his left hand.

"Hey, what did I tell you. He is all intact." I muttered excitedly, "He never had any heart attack; five to seven minutes of cardiorespiratory arrest is bunk."

The doctors were skeptical. Laconic Dr. Zac approached Bobby

PART 2: CALGARY, 1994

in silence; the nurses gave way. He probably realized the truth himself and got down to the business of a full neurological examination. When I left the hospital late in the afternoon, the crowd had dispersed—but a steady stream of visitors went in and out of the room on the neuro floor.

Following twenty-four days of dormancy, Bobby had been reborn, thrusting us into a new set of challenges, even more daunting than the last. The one who facilitated the rebirth was as real as the daylight gleaming at the end of the tunnel, but she never showed up again.

14

LIFE AFTER

JULY 26, 10 A.M. LEFT ARM RESTING OVER HIS HEAD, legs stretched out, Bobby lay on a rollaway bed. His scalp was covered in thinning black hair and a checkerboard, hand drawn with a red pencil. A technologist scooped a bit of clear goop onto a Q-tip, and painstakingly began sticking EEG leads to the coordinates, one at a time, until seventeen were precisely in place.

Bobby seemed to comprehend the meaning of the EEG. He tried to keep still while myoclonus appeared in predictable spurts, causing a slight quivering of his eyelids and minute twitching of his toes. No seizures, though. He looked thin, about forty pounds lighter than he was before the inexplicable coma. Our request for the EEG had been denied until this moment, until Bobby defied death.

It was chaotic early in the morning when I arrived—following the milk run of dropping off Neilly on the main campus for computer camp, and Mon at the Genetics Laboratory in the Health Sciences Centre, where she dissected newborn mice to compare viscera. Bobby was restless, like one of those mice in a cage. His medications were overdue, his breathing laborious. I pressed the button on the wall to show him how to call the nurse on duty, not at all certain if he could grasp the goings-on or focus his eyes to see me clearly. The trachea tube robbed him of his voice.

The nurse pinned the buzzer to the bed sheet and administered nebulized Ventolin. That settled, we began to establish the rudiments of communication—two blinks for "yes" and one for "no." However,

PART 2: CALGARY, 1994

"no" came in other forms as well, like the throwing of arms or legs in displeasure. Bobby's intended actions were preceded by the quivering of his eyes and tremulous hands—like that of an irate flamenco dancer. The flicking limbs predictably lasted a few milliseconds.

Bobby got an extra dose of Clonazepam if he started to seize. He was having a rough time with his trachea; it expelled gobs of mucus, some of which migrated into his mouth through the annular space. The sight and sound of choking and gagging scared us stiff. He was wheezing, though the doctor had said his chest was clear. There wasn't a moment without excitement, a fact that compelled us to stay around. The nurses did rounds and came by once an hour, but Bobby needed constant watching.

The word of his awakening had spread through the hospital like wildfire. A steady stream of doctors, residents, med students, researchers, and ICU nurses traipsed through his room from morning 'til night; it was a teaching hospital, after all. The ward nurses were unhappy—too many visitors. Short of staff, they wanted the family to be there to help, but advised us to limit our numbers to two at a time so they could do their work and our perplexed patient could get a breather.

The neurologists—who couldn't or hadn't helped in the ICU—showed up on their own; even the one who had diagnosed him "decorticate" appeared, red-faced. Some couldn't accept the fact that he had survived the ordeal, and made unyielding comments. "Anoxic patients do not recover full brain function; the cortex damage is permanent."

"The truth is, he never was anoxic," I would rebut. It seemed they didn't know that they had been misled.

THE EEG WAS READ IN RECORD TIME; it was slightly better. The doctors—Mukherjee, Zac, Scott and Bern—all showed up in Bobby's room. As soon as he was a little quiet, meaning seizure free, they said, they would do an MRI of his brain, presumably to discover the extent of the damage done. Even if the MRI results were normal, they warned, enough damage at a molecular level—from letting him seize for a week without the therapeutic dose of anticonvulsants—could keep him from achieving his full potential. We didn't let it get us down. Our hopes were pinned on the opinion of the brain researchers, and not on the old neurologists. They had let us down often enough to destroy our trust.

Sand never visited the neuro ward. His attempt to create a climate of doom had failed.

JULY 29, 1994, 12:00 P.M. WE COULDN'T WAIT for the hospital porter to arrive, or, like so many without family support, Bobby would have missed his urgent appointment. We pushed his wheelchair through a tunnel linking the main building of FHH—where his private room was—to the basement of Baker Cancer Centre, which housed the MRI lab. The long-awaited call for an MRI of Bobby's brain had come with a mundane announcement, following a grueling physio appointment.

Bobby understood what an MRI was and proved it when Bern showed up with Zac in the morning for a clinical test of his intellect and memory. They asked him to tap on his belly if his answer was "Yes," and to do nothing if his answer was "No."

Zac: "Which of the two involve a magnet, CAT scan?"

No tap.

"MRI?"

Tap on belly, with a smile.

Bern: "Are you a medical doctor?"

He raised his eyebrows, meaning, "Yes."

A speech therapist appeared in his room shortly thereafter, with a stack of flash cards bearing similar questions. Until Bobby got tired, he answered them all correctly. And yet he behaved like a toddler, cooperative one moment, defiant the next. He would raise his rear to push himself down the bed in fits of restlessness. Progressively, he became more alert and active as he learned new tricks, but he couldn't sit or stand safely on his own. The nurses tied his left hand to the railing with a strap and kept him in a straitjacket, so he couldn't move. Sad-faced, bewildered in the morning, Bobby was a prisoner for his

PART 2: CALGARY, 1994

own safety. I took the restraints off, worked his stiff hand and leg muscles, and soon he brightened up in appreciation and relief.

Bruce, the wiry old orderly, had a way with this voiceless adult–toddler—a baby just a couple of days before. Skinny but strong for a sixty-year-old, Bruce would transfer Bobby from the bed to the wheelchair with ease and take him for the morning tub bath. Bobby couldn't stand upright. Bruce would motivate him to give his all, a mammoth effort for a silent primate at the dawn of civilization. Following Bobby's bath—dressed in a red T-shirt and black shorts, hair combed uncharacteristically straight back—Bruce would put him back in the wheelchair by making him stand momentarily. But he couldn't keep his head up straight; it would flop forward like a baby's. Bruce refused to give up; his reminders came fast and furious—keep it straight!—until finally he succeeded. Bruce kept us from helping him; Bobby needed to learn to do things for himself.

Speech therapy, physiotherapy and then the call for MRI: it was a dream world for us, a new reality for Bobby. A week before, he had been denied life; now the same hospital was helping him relearn the world—from scratch. Bobby wouldn't know what we had gone through to get him back; he likely wouldn't remember what he was going through to get himself back on his feet. One seldom retains the first few years of experiences of one's life. For Bobby's second childhood, every day seemed like years of progress, but gaps remained that might never be filled.

At the physio sessions, three therapists propped him upright on a wide bench to sit and balance himself on hands placed to his side: a grueling task—huffing, puffing, sweating and fluttering—when relentless myoclonus appeared with predictable frequency, and his weak neck muscles refused to cooperate, keeping his head tilting forward. Thankfully, none of his major muscle groups had suffered atrophy, the reward for our work alongside the nurses and the physiotherapists.

Bobby slept through the MRI session. The chief technologist was cognizant of our ordeal in Montreal and in Calgary. He told us that the MRI looked normal; that is, there was no ischemic injury—caused by lack of blood flow to the brain. The radiologist, Dr. Sevick, confirmed the findings in a terse MRI report in capital letters: "THERE IS NO EVIDENCE OF HYPOXIC ISCHEMIC INJURY[9]."

Finally, the evidence of what we had suspected all along: If a cardiorespiratory arrest of five to seven minutes' duration had ever occurred, its signature would have remained as evidence on the MRI. The clinical history—passed on from JGH to FHH, and that FHH did not verify—was, in fact, false. Diagnostic testing and medications had been denied based on that false information. Had Bobby died as a result, the falsity would have remained as the unchallenged truth.

PART 3:
THUNDER BAY, 2003

15

REALIZATION

JANUARY 9, 2003. THUNDER BAY. The Air Canada flight has landed, and Gale's forehead is pressed tight against the window, sizing up this windswept city of 100,000. A pamphlet is open on my lap, displaying a slogan for tourists: "Naturally Superior." Out in the open, it seems as though a glacier has parted to make room for the runway. Terry Fox ended his journey in this desolate part of Northern Ontario. We are no tourists, nor are we activists. Nonetheless, our journey could end here as well, but before that happens, we must unravel the tangled skein. We check into the Prince Arthur Hotel and take public transport to the Lakehead Psychiatric Hospital (LPH), unannounced in the sub-zero temperatures. Gale is shaking, as much from cold as anxiety. Bobby is broken and broke, disabled and diabetic. Perhaps it is not too late for us to salvage whatever is left; perhaps then we would be able to regard this city as being naturally superior, and not just for its location on the map.

A DIFFERENT KIND OF ANXIETY it was, in July 1994, when Dr. Kimberly, the anesthesiologist, plugged Bobby's trachea tube. He'd tried three days before—with his index finger—forcing Bobby to breathe through his mouth. He couldn't. The tube, originally installed in Montreal, was considerably larger than normal for Bobby's size. Kimberley had to replace it with a new one. It worked well, without irritating his throat. Now we waited with bated breath for him to utter "Mom," "Dad," or similar grown-up words. But the first sound that

PART 3: THUNDER BAY, 2003

emanated from his voice box was a subsonic "Hi," which could easily be misinterpreted without closer scrutiny. Nevertheless, there was no shortage of enthusiasm and experimentation, with his newfound voice generating a multitude of unrecognizable sounds.

Would he be as lippy as he used to be, I wondered as he pointed to his bottom. I buzzed for help. Nurse Cheryl—middle aged, petite but strong—answered the call to facilitate "the big job." Bobby couldn't walk, sit or stand without support, wore Attends for the "little ones." Transferring him, when the sudden movement of any object in front of him caused his legs to buckle, was tricky. You had better be prepared to support his weight. We propped him up, swung his bottom around on the bed so he could step out on the floor and turn, pivoting on one foot, enabling him to provide some support. Cheryl and I provided the rest. He plopped down heavily into the wheelchair. He had started to gain weight, as I had lost mine, through irregular meals, lack of rest and a mountain of stress. Teamwork paid off, and Bobby was transferred successfully to the potty insert. For the second time in his life, he was toilet-trained.

The next morning, his restraints were already removed when I arrived. Nurse Jackie was brushing his teeth for the first time in a month. I wheeled him outside. The trachea tube had been closed for nearly twelve hours. He was trying to talk but no more than a few sounds emerged. Bobby had yet to learn the correct use of his tongue to form words, although his vocal cords seemed intact.

He quickly learned to maneuver his wheelchair with his feet. I took the foot-rests off and asked him to pretend to walk while in the sitting position. He caught on to the idea and learned to move the wheelchair backward and forward unassisted, by pushing or pulling on the floor. Myoclonus and ataxia prevented him from using his hands to grab on to the circular metal push rings attached to the wheels. He began running into walls until I took over and wheeled him out to the terrace garden behind the hospital. The morning sun sparkled on the plush green grass near the sprawling roots of an old birch tree overlooking the slopes of the Canada Olympic Park. The snow-capped mountains on the horizon sparked spiritual thoughts. "Do you like to pray?" I asked. He responded by tightly closing his eyes, facing the mountains. Myoclonus tormented him relentlessly; his eyelids quivered. I sat on the bench next to his wheelchair, knowing that he had understood what I meant.

With visitors restricted, we had more time for ourselves as a family. Bobby was lying on his bed searching for answers, without being able to vocalize the question.

"Do you know what day it is?" I asked. Bewildered, he shook his head from side to side.

"Today is the first of August, 1994; you were injured on June 30, 1994." He closed his eyes in visible pain; tears streamed down onto the pillow. He cried—a voiceless eruption of emotion—the first indication that he was truly awake and that he realized what had happened.

BACK IN THUNDER BAY, GALE NUDGES ME TO HEED the bus driver, who is pointing at an old building ahead on our left. He stops to let us out at a deserted shelter on Algoma Street. In blowing snow, we trudge toward a building. As we get nearer, it takes the shape of a hospital.

16

MILESTONES

LAKEHEAD PSYCHIATRIC HOSPITAL was built in the '30s and expanded in matchbox formation until the '50s. Now, its 500 employees serving 150 beds seem endangered, reminiscent of the old Calgary General Hospital (CGH), which had been shut down and demolished since Bobby was a patient. Dust and debris were hauled away along with memories, and time moved on.

A MONTH HAD GONE BY since Bobby's realization, on that first day of August in 1994, of just what had happened to him. A rehab doctor from CGH assessed him for his impending move from FHH. His mental capacity, attention span and memory were excellent, considering the anaphylactic poisoning and the alleged mistreatment that followed. He sat on his own on the side of his bed without fear of falling, and stood up with assistance. We had taught him to hold the rails and turn his bottom before dangling and resting his feet on the floor. His speech was slurred but improved: he could participate in discussions and voice his opinion. He tried to do more, and as he did, the damage and disorder from the ravages of uncontrolled seizures was unearthed. Myoclonus kept him wheelchair bound. Since I had gone back to work full time at the beginning of the month, he had made improvements, but none came without struggle. I had several projects on the go in various geographic locations—Pittsburgh, Edmonton, Montreal and Toronto. My boss had pinch-hit in my absence, or I would have had no job to go back to. Soon, I became immersed in a stack of backlogged items during the day that left me working with Bobby at FHH at night, well past visiting hours. Gale and I would interact during our shift overlap. She would be on her way home, after attending to Bobby's therapies and mealtimes through the day.

The trachea tube came out completely in August 1994, plug and all. There were no stitches, simply a piece of tape over the opening in his throat—it would heal on its own. Physio and speech therapy sessions went on as usual, though Bobby couldn't do much of anything for gasping, coughing and wheezing. Breathing had been easier through the tube—the path of least resistance—than through his mouth. However, he could balance himself better and sit erect.

Bobby wanted to go out the moment Gale had left for the day. "That's not the way to the garden," I said, when he pointed to "B" on the elevator panel. But he insisted: basement. "Now where?" I asked impatiently. He turned his head to the arrow on the wall—*Health Sciences Centre*. I didn't know the way through the tunnel, or if there was wheelchair access.

Irrepressible, he tried hard to talk, producing a multitude of mysterious sounds, but nothing comprehensible. Through silent words and flamenco gestures, he convinced me that he would show me the way around the complex by pointing. I pushed his wheelchair through the security area of the tunnel, changing direction several times along the way. We went up the elevator in the research building, down the hallway, down another set of elevators from the second floor to the first, down the hallway around the staff lounge to a large hallway by the statue of Hippocrates, and finally to the Bach Centre. He remembered; his old memory was largely intact.

The next day, Gale was all smiles. She couldn't wait to tell me that Bobby had walked three steps at physiotherapy—with assistance. Essentially, he could now stand up and balance himself. Walking would follow naturally. But he wouldn't wait; he wanted to visit the med school again, and asked for prophylactic puffs of Ventolin. Reluctantly, I wheeled him to the Bach Centre, where he once again demonstrated to himself that he remembered everything, and displayed no patience if I took a wrong turn.

PART 3: THUNDER BAY, 2003

The *Calgary Herald* published his story again: "Doctor out of Coma." More visitors showed up in his hospital room on the tenth floor—high school friends, debate partners, teachers, professors, people we knew, people we didn't and had never met, and Jen. She hadn't been visible during our battle to reinstate medications, but no sooner had Bobby come out of the coma than she thrust herself into the scene.

JEN'S APPEARANCE WAS A HARBINGER OF TROUBLE. Snippets of information emerged by osmosis. During family meetings at the hospital, Gale often questioned what had happened on Day Zero. "Western foods do not have nuts except for desserts or cookies," she would wonder. "Chinese food is nearly the same, but Thai food is another matter. But Bobby didn't go there." Jen's appearance justified our work in shifts to help with patient care, but more importantly, to keep Bobby out of harm's way—especially at meal times. Bobby's deposition in December 1997 under questioning from the lead defense counsel, Mart, confirmed our concerns:

Mart: What had happened, as best you can recall, leading to the 1993 hospitalization?[10]

Bob: What happened was Jen and I were eating dinner—or attempting to eat dinner at Buchanan's [restaurant in Calgary]. Apparently, Jen had some soup and I had another appetizer. Jen said, Why don't you try my soup? And I tried a bit of her soup and I got a reaction to it right away.

SOON AFTER, THE NIGHT NURSE reported verbally, and recorded in the charts, Jen had visited Bobby's room from 12:00 midnight to 4:00 A.M. and kept the lights on—"reading." The nurse also mentioned the dreaded word: "seizures." I called and met with the hospital security. Had Jen been using her mother's physician pass to gain access, they wondered. Otherwise, she would have been caught. No visitor was authorized in a patient's room in the dead of night. However, the hospital administration, for reasons unknown at the time, wanted her visits to continue, but during the visiting hours, and for no more than an hour and a half:

Mart: You had discussed marriage with her, but no plans had been made?
Bob: We had discussed many things. She had brought them up. She had brought up marriage, she had brought up children, she had brought up naming children. We were careful not to be—. We kind of drifted after my acceptance to McGill, and were more non-committal to each other. And the drive was a fun, almost a goodbye trip, and we would see how things would go after that.
Mart: Are you talking about the drive across Canada in late June?
Bob: Correct.
Mart: Had you suggested that it would be best to end the relationship at that time?
Bob: In August I did.
Mart: August of 1990.
Bob: Four.
Mart: —four?
Bob: She was seeing a psychiatrist afterwards.
Mart: After August 1994?
Bob: No, after the incident in Montreal, she had begun seeing a psychiatrist, and I advised her that, you know, it's going to be difficult, that perhaps it's in her best interest to end our relationship.
Mart: This had been a serious relationship prior to the incident in 1994?
Bob: How do you define "serious"?
Mart: She was your girlfriend for some period of time?
Bob: Yes.
Mart: You had lived together?
Bob: No.

PART 3: THUNDER BAY, 2003

The nocturnal visits stopped, but the falsehoods spread. Jen had apparently told the Montreal police[11] that she'd been living with Bobby in Montreal from June 23, 1994. A trail of purchases in Alberta up until their departure from Calgary on June 25, 1994, proved otherwise. Others were told, presumably by Jen, that "Bobby had poisoned himself."

Meanwhile, Bobby passed another milestone. The dietitian or the nurse had been infusing 300 cc of Jevity tube-feed directly into his stomach six times a day. That was his food. For drinks, they would water flush the NG tube routinely and weigh him on a scale. The synthetic food made no contact with his taste buds. All of that changed one day when he pulled out the NG tube halfway. The ward nurse Gene pulled it out the rest of the way and refused to put it back; it was causing a lot of pain. What a difference when Mon and I walked in the next morning! Janice was feeding Bobby his breakfast by mouth, half a teaspoon at a time. He could taste the difference between peach yogurt and cream of wheat; the cream of wheat remained nearly untouched.

As exciting as this was, Bobby's newfound experiments with taste couldn't go on without a swallow test. Gale and I anxiously waited by the 4th floor radiology department later in the morning, failing to understand why such a test would be necessary when Bobby had swallowed food already. The therapist—about to give him a cookie to start the test—was startled when both of us jumped out of our chairs in panic: "What are the ingredients of the cookie?" She didn't know. The triumph nearly brought tragedy.

The swallow test went ahead without the deadly cookies, but our anxiety remained. Gale took the dietitian aside and alerted her to Bobby's allergies—not just peanuts, but nuts of any kind. We complained about the breakfast peanut butter packages that showed up in the lunchroom by the fridge, where food and drinks were kept. I took pains to throw them out in the morning, but larger quantities appeared the next day.

Two nurses knocked on the closed door at shift overlap, interrupting our conversation to let us know that Jen wanted to see Bobby.

The shift overlap meeting wasn't about the progress Bobby made day to day, although he'd made plenty. It was about Jen showing up at all hours of the day or night, especially during Gale's shifts, offering comments on Bobby's "nine lives."

"She can't come in," we said in chorus. She sent in Pat, the nurse in charge, to break up the meeting.

Jen returned again that evening, while Bobby's high school classmates, Koshif and Peter, were assisting with a walk around the ward. At my wit's end, frustration took over my better judgment. I told her to go to hell and leave us alone. It had dawned on us that someone in the hospital administration could be behind her activities. Gale had warned against allowing myself to be provoked. "Our focus is for Bobby to get better," she reminded me. "Nothing else matters." She'd had a run-in with Jen days before, when she showed up at lunchtime. Dr. Field had had to put Bobby on a systemic steroid for the next three days to combat a perfume-induced asthma attack that didn't respond to puffs. The need for us to become Bobby's legal guardians surfaced again.

The next afternoon, I asked the director of nursing, Gene, to get Jen off our backs. She wanted to get together with Marg and talk to Bobby. But Bobby was in no shape to judge. He was searching in the darkness of his memory for what had happened, from the time of the poisoning to this day. His speech was nearly formed, but slurred, rambling and loud. He had asked Mon to name the doctors who had given up on him, and what those doctors had told us about his prognosis. Overwhelmed by the increasing number of visitors that showed up in his room during normal visiting hours—with a variety of questions, interests and motives—frustrations overtook him at times, demanding more attention from us.

Two nurses from the ICU visited and shared "privileged" information with Bobby, whom they considered a doctor. It was unbelievable that he had survived the ordeal, they said. "ICU routinely snuffs out patients they think will not survive, or will survive in a PVS, at the discretion of the ICU chief." It seemed that few ever found this out; patient

PART 3: THUNDER BAY, 2003

confidentiality, which keeps this information behind an iron curtain, is simply a cover; privacy is a double-edged sword. The reputation of the institution overrides ethics; color and cologne cover the taint.

A HOSPITAL IS NEVER A PARADISE, nor a devil's den. It is a place of trust, holding the most valuable of all worldly possessions. Once that trust is shattered, it becomes a paradigm of distrust. But now, in 2003, Bobby is not a patient here at LPH in Thunder Bay; he is a new doctor, at the bottom of the totem pole—a fellow in psychiatry. Allison, the department secretary, takes us into his well-furnished, comfortable office. Suppressing surprise but appearing happy, Bobby greets us and introduces us—to the people around the basement outpatient clinic and to the office staff, without hesitation—as his parents.

This hasn't happened since February 8, 1999.

17

STEALTH MOVE

BOBBY WALKS REASONABLY WELL IN THUNDER BAY, along the long lonely corridors of LPH. He has doffed his dead wheelchair—batteries don't hold charge. We follow him into the waiting elevator as he presses a bare button on the panel, turns his head, and empties his lungs. "Doctor's residence is on the third, unmarked for extra security." We go through a nondescript, locked double door into a long and wide hallway that loops back into a common kitchen at the entrance. A dozen dark, spacious, empty rooms seem to jut into the rectangular hallway like echo chambers. They haven't seen an occupant in ages, or so it appears, and none is here now besides Bobby. He's picked the room closest to the kitchen, by the double doors. His luggage is strewn over the floor, as if someone had dropped a load of cargo and left in a hurry. He must carry his keys, pager, and cell phone on him at all times, to function during and after hours, and to pass through half a dozen or so locked doors between his office and the residence. He moved here on Monday, January 5, 2003, after an overnight stay at the same hotel Gale and I checked into last night. He has to be on his feet whenever he goes anywhere. This tires him immensely, but Bobby perseveres. He has no other option. He is guarded in asking for things, lest his new employer should come to know his story.

BACK IN FHH, NOBODY WAS WILLING TO SAY THAT HE'D EVER walk again, but his walking progressed, aided, from three to six to sixty-six steps, and he was eager to show off to Helen, an old friend,

PART 3: THUNDER BAY, 2003

by walking all the way around the entire neuro floor. He remembered having lunch with her on June 24, 1994, the day before leaving Calgary. Helen and I held his hand on either side, while Jessica pushed his wheelchair a step behind, in case his legs buckled. He attempted the walk unaided. His gait resembled that of a child. His left leg would occasionally misstep from the onset of myoclonus, and the perception of even the slightest sudden movement through the corner of his eyes made him nearly collapse like a soldier taking a direct hit. The girls urged him to stop.

Jessica's father Abraham was being stitched in the ER for a nasty cut to his hand. I wheeled Bobby in to visit him. In the waiting room, a *Maclean*'s magazine displayed news of O.J. Simpson's trial. That seemed more interesting to Bobby than visiting; he could turn pages, something he hadn't been able to do the day before.

All heads turned in the direction of a sudden thud. Jessica, a serious med student who did clinic all day, had crashed to the floor, unconscious. Moments before, she had been sitting on a chair, her head resting on a desk. No one realized that she was tired and dehydrated. The impact of the O.J. story on Bobby was striking; it made him appear indifferent—uncaring even—about Jessica and her father. With little empathy, he remarked, "She'll be all right." She was, and as I wheeled him back to the ward, it occurred to Bobby that neither Nicole Brown Simpson nor Ronald Goldman were anaphylactic, or O.J. wouldn't have needed to use gloves to cover up what he had done.

Marg Haynes—a social psychologist and faith-touch healer—came at night to work with Bobby. On his bed with bent knees, Bobby did pushups, his first since his injuries. He could turn over on his stomach to push himself up, demonstrating a formidable tenacity to get better, dispelling Jen's apparent assertion that "Bobby did it to himself."

Despite haunting disturbances, progress was made. Each night, the nurse would administer the last dose of medication of the night and turn off the lights, keeping the buzzer pinned next to Bobby's pillow. Straitjackets, hand restraints and Attends were things of the past, as were Bobby's inhibitions. He could buzz for help, and if necessary, ask for Ventolin or Tylenol. These days weren't without scares, however. A major aspiration was averted on a day that started with an early bath, a good breakfast, and a major choking spell brought on by a Tylenol elixir, causing him to throw up.

Albert, a Calgary businessman with a wife and three small children, wasn't so lucky. His gall bladder operation had been successful, but he was left unattended post-surgery. He'd had a major aspiration that nearly drowned him in his own vomit. The incident left Albert severely brain injured, and a long-term patient of unit 101.

Bobby started to develop a disdain for the doctors who had given up on him. It was his turn to get even. He gave nicknames to all the doctors on the floor:

"There goes Dr. Rabbit."

"That's not Dr. Rabbit; that's Dr. Fox."

"Always in a hurry . . . prescribes medications . . . doesn't read chart."

He'd invite everyone to play chess with him. He played with Bern, the neuro resident, and won a can of pop that he kept unopened to display as a souvenir.

Bobby used his rediscovered verbal skills, however impeded by slurring, to befriend the staff—nurses, physiotherapist, occupational therapist, speech therapist and recreational therapist. To survive in a high-patient-ratio hospital, he took to addressing them individually. "How is my goddess today?" They seemed to like sharing a laugh or two with this "compliant and amiable" patient.

"Things are favorable; physical matters such as motor control, balance, etc. continue to improve for three months," Dr. Mukherjee explained as he examined Bobby. "Intelligence [cognitive functions], such as speech and language, continue to improve for 18 months. As far as physical signs, such as posturing of body parts, they are tone related." He was not optimistic about "graceful movement and fluidity," but "strength, coordination and spasticity" would improve with time.

Bobby appeared mentally competent, but deficits in reading, writing, concentration, basic math skills, emotional intelligence (EQ) and judgment were revealed as time progressed. Physically, he could put

PART 3: THUNDER BAY, 2003

on his glasses and eat a few spoonfuls of food, though the onset of myoclonus could turn the spoon into a rocket on a flight to the ceiling. Progressive attempts yielded better results, but spills were unavoidable.

At shift overlap, Gale told me that Bern had mentioned to her that they would arrange a psychologist or a social worker to help Bobby deal with his emotional concerns.

"Bobby isn't a psychiatric patient," I replied. Our experiences with psychiatrists, social workers and psychologists—Psych, Sow and Psy, as Bobby called them—had been wretchedly negative, starting with Jen's mother.

The hospital ordered Bobby's neuropsychological evaluation—grueling tests that lasted six hours and stretched over two days. It was necessary to ascertain the damage wrought by the injuries he sustained, but the timing was interesting: it coincided with Bobby's willingness to allow us to become his guardians so long as he was in the hospital. The issue had been with us almost since the beginning, when we realized that hospital ethics was nothing more than window dressing, and social work, within the confines of a hospital, was an exercise in public relations. We broached the subject soon after Bobby was able to understand, that someone as vulnerable as he was needed a voice, a voice other than his own.

The test results came in. They focused on family relationships: "Dr. C— is right-handed. His father had insisted he use his right hand as a child, and it is possible he might otherwise have been left-handed or ambidextrous."

"That is false," Gale said. "Besides, what does this have to do with Bobby's current level of intelligence?" It had everything to do with the position the hospital would take in opposing guardianship. They appeared horrified at that thought, something that alerted my suspicion of serious wrongdoing. They had noticed that I was keeping contemporaneous notes.

IN THE EARLY MORNING OF SEPTEMBER 13, 1994, BOBBY was moved to the Calgary General Hospital in an ambulance, before I could arrive at FHH to accompany him. I was scheduled to be there to participate in the move. The reason for the earlier departure time became obvious when I examined the discharge papers[13] prepared by a fourth-year resident we'd never seen in the ICU. "Over the course of Bobby's stay in the Foothills ICU," she wrote, "there were numerous difficulties in dealing with his family . . . the family was unable to accept Bobby's prognosis and was very difficult to deal with." Nonetheless, she confirmed that Bobby had eaten in a Chinese restaurant. She made no mention of the MRI results that refuted the false clinical history.

I left FHH around 9 A.M., with little information as to where Bobby would be at the CGH. I left the car parked on a far street to avoid the menace of no-parking signs, and ran up the grassy embankment through the overfilled parking lot into the rear entrance of the hospital. It was a large, dated, inner city building, located in the northeast corner of the city in an old neighborhood, five minutes from the P-C Centre in good traffic. It had grown like a massive organism over the years. The add-ons of different vintages, now stuck together, looked spooky and felt downright depressing. The entrails of the basement hallways of the old H block led through the G block that joined the newer M block with a long ramp. In the maze, I finally found Bobby in H Block, in a room shared with three other patients. No one knew him, except through charts, which few read.

The head nurse and the attending showed us around the facilities. CGH was not a teaching hospital. It appeared to have fewer politics, and a staff that could focus more on treating patients than on treating patients as teaching objects. Bobby and I met with Dr. McGovern—the physiatrist, doctor of physical medicine—a rehab doc. Her message was clear: they did not have sufficient staff or funds to care for the patients and therefore depended on families to look after their needs such as bath, feeding, and general care. For those without family support, a bath was given twice a week. The patients were encouraged to be independent and help themselves. For the first time in our hospital experience, the need for family was emphasized at the care level. The nurses' role was to administer medications that doctors ordered,

PART 3: THUNDER BAY, 2003

general facilitation and patient management. Their goal was to clear out long-term patients from the hospital to the outside world. Patients were scheduled to participate in therapies. Bobby was to undergo a rehab program for the brain-injured for the ensuing month.

CGH PRESENTED A NEW SET OF OBSTACLES and opportunities. For one, Gale could not drive cross-town to feed Bobby after Neilly's school had started. Since the hospital was near my work, the task fell to me to rush over, brown bag in hand, to help him eat, have my lunch at the same time, and then rush back to my work. By the time I'd arrive at CGH, Bobby would be sitting in his chair waiting, his lunch tray in front of him already. Some days he would venture to help himself, but the tray would refuse to cooperate and drop on the floor. In his quivering voice, muffled by guilt, he would say, "Oh well, there goes another." I would hurry downstairs to the kitchen and get him a replacement, making sure there was no contamination from nuts of any kind.

At times, I watched him stuff nearly half of my sandwich into his mouth all at once. Feigning anger I would say, "What did you do that for?", knowing full well that the meager hospital food hardly satisfied his hunger. The drug Epival made him ravenous. In the evening after work, I would visit to help with dinner and give him his bath. On some weekends, I would take him home on a day pass, and let him crawl on the carpet like a toddler. He would get up on his own, holding the rails that I'd put up throughout the house, and walk, holding my hands, and go up or down the stairs.

NOW AT LPH, NEARLY NINE YEARS HAVE PASSED. In this remote northern Ontario city, Bobby is without support of any kind. It's eerie to meet the chief psychiatrist—congenial, in her fifties—late in the evening as she comes by, while we wait in an adjacent office for Bobby's door to open, and him to emerge from his patient-related paperwork and consultation. We expected to see no one in the basement outpatient clinic. We are even more surprised when she asks, "What does he need?"

We have been asking around for sources of support in the community; the words may have reached her ears. Since his move, Bobby has been doing everything by himself and getting very tired. People in the hospital have been noticing. Toronto—where he moved from after completing his residency training at the Clarke Institute of Psychiatry—offered help to get him up and get him going in the morning. Nothing is set up here, and that is a serious challenge to his well-being. It seems just a matter of time before he gets too sick to function. Though the atmosphere in the lonely quarters is depressing, the few staff that are here appear to be accommodating and friendly.

"He would probably say he doesn't need any help," I reply.

"That's what he said to us when he was here last December. We could have set it all up for him if he said he needed the help."

Bobby didn't want to ask for help. He didn't want to risk being rejected. He needed the job, desperately. He didn't want to expose all his afflictions, assuming someone else—his references—hadn't told her already. Too much has happened for Gale and me to know where things stand. We can tell he needs help, and money, but how badly broke he is, we haven't a clue. Looking at each other, we can't help but wonder what happened to the money he received in settlement. Yet another mystery to solve.

18

LIFTING FOG

"GO AS FAR AWAY AS POSSIBLE," the lawyers had told him. To our shock and horror, Bobby obeyed and cut off ties from us the day he signed on the dotted line, on February 8, 1999. He left Calgary. For the past four years, the lawyers have had the power to control him—and they have done so to the point where all his money has vanished. His adviser at the Clarke had told him to move to Thunder Bay—where he could focus, away from all the distractions, and prepare for the upcoming Royal College exam. Ironically, he probably doesn't have the money to pay the fees. Bobby is now banished to this remote city, penniless, away from support—one of the conditions of the settlement to keep us in the dark. Like us, he is thinking, wondering whether or where to begin. I can see that he is searching, as are we all.

IT WAS A DIFFERENT SEARCH for Bobby at CGH. Was Jen innocent, or, had she played a role in that gruesome night? Should he believe the hospital—who were sold on her sob story—or his parents? For the brain injured, whose memory of the trauma is often erased by the lingering shadow of a coma, "truth" presents a difficult dilemma. Should Bobby listen to the hospital social worker, who was wooing him as a friend, or the family that took him home on weekends, and most weeknights, and waited on him, hand and foot, to get him better? He wasn't sure who to believe, now that he was making progress. Like a toddler torn between toxic toys and parental warnings, he called Jen to visit him at the CGH.

MEDICAL MALADY

He wanted to go back to Montreal to reclaim his neurology residency position. Although he'd been declared decorticate, his medical knowledge remained intact. He thought I would set him up in Montreal, just like I had the last time. His disabilities didn't enter into his mind. For me, however, providing care and support that Bobby needed made return to Montreal a near impossibility.

An idea crossed our collective thoughts. If months of intense therapy could build his energy level up to the point where he could handle the rigors of residency, Bobby could start his medicine rotation in Calgary, as an exchange resident from Montreal. It wasn't to be; Calgary wrote him off, and the MNI, who wanted to see him function up close, would have nothing to do with the idea.

Bobby was disappointed, yet persistent. He was putting the cart of his career before the horse of recovery. He argued, "If I miss this year, I will have to go through the Canadian Resident Matching[14] again, and who will help me then?"

To prove that he could handle his return to Montreal, he wanted to take part in the Terry Fox run, a mere four days away. The idea was spawned in FHH as a way to denounce those doctors who'd given up on him. He collected over $200 in pledges from doctors, nurses and friends.

"Why do you want to do this?" I asked.

His reply was simple. "I took part in it every year for the last six years—that's why." Indeed, he was the recipient of the Terry Fox Humanitarian award of 1989.

A reporter once wrote[15], "His early exposures to hospital led Bobby to volunteer at the Alberta Children's Hospital, where he spends most Sundays in the emergency ward, calming the fears of young patients, entering their world through his hand puppet, Tom the Cow."

Bobby walked the Terry Fox run, assisted, on September 18, 1994, at North Glenmore Park; all five kilometers of it. He was wobbly at first on the rough pavement, but refused to sit down on his wheelchair, even though he fell once on 66th Street and scraped his knee. He got up and kept on walking. Gale, Neilly and my boss took turns

PART 3: THUNDER BAY, 2003

helping, while one of us kept his wheelchair close behind, just in case the unforeseen happened. It didn't. Long training walks in the entrails of the hospital between buildings F and M had helped him build up his endurance. Going up and down the stairs holding rails had improved his coordination and balance. That, topped up with a few road sessions before the event, made success possible.

Not surprisingly, Jen came and met his roommate patients: George, 84, a writer–painter with a neck injury from a mild stroke that had caused him to fall down the basement stairs in his home; John, 64, an MS patient, diabetic and paralyzed from the waist down; and Steve, 17, paralyzed from the shoulder blade down. He was wheelchair bound with multiple internal injuries. A drunk driver had crossed over the median and crashed into the vehicle he was driving, instantly killing his mother, who was in the passenger seat.

George was impressed with the "girlfriend." "Oh, a psychiatrist's daughter," he quipped. "A medical resident as well!" John was skeptical of her story—that Bobby had harmed himself—and displayed ambivalence. Steve, having heard that Bobby was severely allergic to peanuts, felt guilty keeping chocolate-coated peanuts and chocolate bars in his drawer and under his pillow. He didn't want to eat peanuts in the same room as Bobby, and asked to be transferred to another. The nurse moved Steve to the room with Keith. Keith, 45, had fallen off a bike, and as he fell, he went over a bridge and hit a boulder on the ground twenty feet below. He suffered a hip fracture and multiple internal injuries. Keith and Bobby became friends, providing support for each other.

Two days later, George left and wished Bobby as long a life as his own. John remained remarkably self-sufficient, considering he had no use of his legs. I couldn't help but compare Bobby's predicament with those of the other rehabilitants, but it was futile. Poisoning and a multitude of mistreatments set him apart. However, comparing the diligence of a 17-year-old with that of the medical student opened up questions only Jen could answer, and Bobby wanted them answered:

MEDICAL MALADY

Mart: Why did you sue Jen—?[16]
Bob: I wanted to know what happened on the night–or on the day of June 30th, 1994, as well as what her knowledge was during the time I was in a coma.
Mart: Did you not ask her that prior to issuing a Statement of Claim against her?
Bob: She wished not to talk to me [about Day Zero].
Mart: So you never asked her about what happened on June 30th?
Bob: How could I ask her if she wouldn't talk to me?

Bobby called me at work—from where, I didn't know for sure—to tell me that he was out of the hospital. A female medical student had taken him out in the afternoon, without signing for it. He wanted to hear for himself how the peanuts went into his mouth on Day Zero. Knowing the dangers, I pleaded with him to focus on his therapy. The hospital was pushing him to be independent and to leave, notwithstanding his drug levels were still being adjusted, and that his recovery score was 3.5 to 4 on a scale of 0 to 7, 7 being normal.

He returned to the hospital late at night. The next day there were two messages on my answering machine: Bobby's medications were being increased, and he wasn't going out any more. He was gravely ill. He had a fever, wheezed through the night, and went for chest physiotherapy in the morning to dislodge lung congestion. Whatever he had been exposed to on his outing had caused a severe reaction. The consequence was a toxic regression: the clarity of his speech worsened (dysarthria), his voice was hoarse, he was back on intravenous steroid—Salumedrol—given to patients in severe allergic reaction or anaphylaxis. They administered nebulized Pulmacort and Ventolin together every two hours. The resident, Dr. Demchuck, began reducing one of his anticonvulsants that interacted with the allergy medications that spiked myoclonus.

Three days passed, and Bobby's temperature remained in the 38.5 to 40°C range. He received no antipyretic. I asked for the doctor

PART 3: THUNDER BAY, 2003

on-call to give him medication to bring the fever under control. She snapped, "I am the doctor here; it is my decision." She refused to intervene without consulting a neurologist. I requested an alternate doctor. The hospital advised that a family physician with privileges at CGH would be acceptable. Dr. Kennedy, an allergy specialist we knew, came and gave him Tylenol. The fever eased to 37.1°C, and Bobby felt better by noon. The fog of coma seemed to be lifting—ever so slowly—with the realization that he'd stepped back into the minefield, and miraculously survived, again.

BUT WOULD HE SURVIVE HERE AT LPH? Bobby's appointment isn't confirmed yet, and he's not sure when he is getting paid, if at all. We walk to the nurse's station through a narrow corridor some distance away, where his food tray is delivered and waiting to be picked up. He is essentially living on charity from the hospital, for now.

19

LAST HAUNT

I CARRY THE FOOD TRAY BACK to the doctor's quarters—Bobby's hands are still unsteady. He follows me to the kitchenette and sits heavily on one of the wooden chairs. For the first time in four years, I can sit down and talk to him face to face, and get some answers.

"I can't believe what happened to you," I say, resting the tray on the table in front of him.

"Well, I am still alive. Wasn't I worth saving?" His head hanging low, he inspects the meager food on the plate, as I lift the round metal cover with a hole in the middle.

"Of course! But look what they did to you; the scumbags got rich at our expense. Why did you listen?"

"I was caught in a tangled skein, like a fly in a web," Bobby replies. "I couldn't see my way around."

There were efforts all along to isolate him, an alienation process that began in the early stages of his recovery. He is afraid, afraid for his life, although when I ask, he says no, no one is threatening him. But when Gale visited his apartment soon after the settlement, she found Balinese (peanut) sauce; a stark reminder of what could happen.

WEDNESDAY, OCTOBER 26, 1994. A PHYSIATRIST, Dr. Barton, had left an urgent voice message for me at work. Bobby had fallen at 9:30 A.M., face down, fractured his nose, and suffered a concussion. "Damn it." I slammed the file drawer in frustration and rushed off to the

PART 3: THUNDER BAY, 2003

hospital. There had been six incidents reports already, five of lesser consequence. This should have jarred their conscience to adopt, at our request, a safety helmet policy. We had bought a safety helmet for Bobby when he was a child learning to skate and play hockey. Workers in factories wear them, so do bikers on the street. Why aren't seizure-prone patients required to wear them in physiotherapy? The hospital had ignored our request; it was a matter of individual choice, they said. But the individual was post-coma—recovering "like a house on fire" in many aspects, but still like a preadolescent child.

Another serious head injury made the argument for guardianship stronger, so long as Bobby remained in the hospital. He had already given us permission. A legal guardian would have a voice in his treatment; parents of adult patients have none. The hospital social worker tried to convince Bobby to denounce the plan, claiming that we wanted power over him. Such nonsense. They declared that Bobby's concussions were our fault! The hospital administration—the head nurse, the psychiatrist, VP Administration, VP patient care, the family counselor and others—met with Bobby alone. Bobby was amused. "Each one of the participants took aim at the parents," he relayed. The CGH and FHH administrations were linked through the Calgary Regional Health Authority, CRHA.

The social worker—Sow, abbreviated Bobby—took him to the downtown unemployment office, skipping therapy sessions. She counseled him on "independent living" with social assistance in a halfway house, or with friends. She had little use for patient history, or the patient's needs and aspirations, just so long as he was away from his family. She offered incentives: the hospital would pay for specialty drugs and Handibus tickets if he'd stay in an outpatient hostel. She would continue to help him with his "spirituality."

Bobby announced that a new psychologist had seen him lately. She referred to Jen as his "girlfriend" and suggested we were to blame for his "illness." The pressure of alienation intensified as time progressed. He would hardly greet us, and if he did, it was "Hey," and then he would clam up. On hold were the usual "Hi Dad," or, "Hi Mom," that preceded the day's goings on. Whatever emotions were left in him post coma were being chipped away with each passing psy session, tearing the notion of family from his psyche.

Following the advice of the Association for Rehabilitation of the Brain Injured, and Southern Alberta Brain Injury Society— "Administration is too powerful, fighting the system (to improve safety and treatment) would be futile; it could tear family apart at the expense of the patient; let them get their way"— Gale and I dropped the guardianship application.

Dr. McGovern, the physiatrist, stayed above the patient-control fray and took over the head injury patients halfway through Bobby's hospital stay. Patient interest alone was in her mind, and in the mind of the neurologist. The neurology resident who'd researched his drug interaction was about to leave. Bobby became more wobbly, even with a higher dose of the anti-myoclonic drug. He was disappointed that no one would monitor his neurologic progress in close proximity. It was tricky titrating the tyranny of twin disorders: epilepsy and myoclonus. Any rapid change in medication threatened a tsunami of seizures that caused setbacks when recovery was supposed to be rapid, ahead of the anticipated plateau—a narrow window post coma.

Clonazepam increased, Tegretol reduced, Prednisone phased out, antibiotic in its last dose, Bobby had vastly improved control of his myoclonus. He could speak at 180 syllables a minute and walk around obstacles. Still, the latest serious allergic reaction and the drug interaction cost him valuable recovery time.

The neurologist introduced Piracetam, from Belgium, apparently a wonder drug. With the drug interaction dealt with, and the "girlfriend" a haunting history—since he went out with Jen looking for answers and got a severe allergic reaction instead—Bobby made quantum progress. On November 25, 1994, I brought him home for an overnight stay, his first in five months. He walked with a walker, slept in his own bed and sang in his booming voice: "It was just a dream . . ."

He showed off his new improved handwriting—no longer a nest of oblong scribbles and twitchy spikes, but recognizable letters that made up real words. The drugs were working, and he worked even

PART 3: THUNDER BAY, 2003

harder. He had been asking the resident to increase the dosages to speed up his progress, and pulling rank as a doctor to get it. Now he could lift a glass of orange juice—or a cup of coffee from the dinner table—with one hand, and take a sip or two in loud slurps, to let the world know that he no longer needed straws. I didn't need to be on the alert to catch a flying glass from midair like an outfielder, and be prepared to get a sticky cold shower in the process.

FRIDAY, JANUARY 20, 1995. AN ORDEAL THAT HAD TAKEN US TO three hospitals in two provinces, over seven long months of defying death to pursue life, had paid off. Beating all odds, Bobby came home, and with him an accumulation of belongings that had grown from a single blue apron and a white sheet to a carload of presents and the memory of murderous notations in his chart: "decorticate," "the chance for recovery to a meaningful functional state is nil."

Discharge from the rehab hospital was unceremonious—indeed uneventful—but it was a giant step in getting back to a semblance of normalcy. Dr. McGovern had left out all matters unrelated to the diagnosis and treatment of our patient from the discharge summary. It contained no falsehood, amplifying the difference between the discharge summary of a resident in a teaching hospital and one written by a professional in a treating hospital.

A month before Bobby's release, Dr. McGovern had arranged a family conference with therapists—speech therapist, occupational therapist and physiotherapist. With Sow conspicuously absent, so was any mention of independent living away from home. The therapists commented on Bobby's progress—control of gait and performance, Jefferson hand function test, computer training, reading rate, articulation—and life post-hospital. He would work with a neurologist to become accustomed to medical work, and in an unexpected hook, he was to visit the Psy at FHH, to which he didn't say no.

JANUARY 11, 2003. BACK AT LPH, I ATTEMPT TO SQUEEZE FOUR years of conversations into one weekend. For that long, we have been virtually cut off, insulated by people we hardly knew. Bobby hasn't talked to me about anything substantive since the day I brought him back from the judicial dispute resolution (JDR) in Calgary. I describe the elaborate hooks and schemes that were obvious to us, but to which he was oblivious. His injured mind—washed in a multitude of psy-psych sessions, tested and retested in numerous neuropsych challenges, trowelled by adverse counseling—had lost its luster of sharpness.

I say, "If the doctors had been smart, they would have admitted to their mistakes, and cut the legal mullahs out."

"That's not the way it goes."

"The complication was the girl; it wasn't just a matter of multiple mistakes."

"I was in a coma, and since then . . ." He pauses to take a puff of medication, and I take the opportunity to clear the table.

"You can't remember. Let me take you back to Montreal, see if you can." I return to the chair. "My words are verifiable truth; I've kept my diary and all the files." More often than not, authorities—doctors and lawyers in positions of trust and power—create works of fiction to drown out the voices of truth and submerge their murderous mistakes in the murky waters of healthcare, and then hide behind the curtain of confidentiality.

PART 4:
MONTREAL, 1995

20

RETURN

MAY 30, 1995. FLIGHT AC-144 TOOK OFF from Calgary on time. The first two passengers with economy-class boarding passes were ushered in, long before flight time, to adjacent business-class seats at the bulkhead. The stewardess took one look at the younger passenger's face and decided not to put him in economy; the flight wasn't full. That was our first lucky break following a disastrous start.

If she had seen him a few days before, she might have fainted or summoned security. He sported a ponytail, black bushy beard and nails that had grown since Day Zero. It was a look that he'd steadfastly hung on to—one that gave him the appearance of a swashbuckling pirate with multiple war wounds—until he received a letter from Dr. Francis at the MNI, offering the commencement of his residency training. Supriya, a Calgary medical resident he admired, took him to a coiffeuse, whose work exposed the bumps and bruises from numerous falls, fractures and concussions that decorated his otherwise handsome face. Now he looked clean cut, and his manners improved with his new image. But he needed time, time to hold people's attention for the first few minutes, so they wouldn't dismiss him as drunk or intellectually challenged, listening to his slurred, halting speech. Once the initial contact was made and the situation explained, he could handle conversations with ease. Bobby would be observed in Montreal for three to six months, and if he could handle the workload, they would let him go on to complete the program in neurology.

PART 4: MONTREAL, 1995

Earlier that morning, the Chinook wind had been pushing hard at the crimson edge of the dark cloud toward the brown haze in the eastern horizon, revealing the "Jewel of the West" through an umbrella of poplar trees beyond Glenmore Lake. "Daaad, have you called La Tour?"

He meant La Tour Belvedere, an apartment hotel in Montreal. My chain of thought, of what had happened to Bobby since we'd moved to this city of high expectations, and what would happen to him now and to the rest of our family, was interrupted. I wanted to yell, "Go back to sleep; it's too early; we aren't leaving yet." Instead, I said, "You'd better let me have the binder." The binder was our bible—it contained not only the telephone number for La Tour, but all other information I had put together to help Bobby survive in Montreal.

Bobby had probably stayed up all night in the excitement of returning to Montreal. I hadn't had much sleep either, for all the worries. I took a glance at the bedroom clock and walked into his room to get the binder. He gripped the "Saskipole" with his left hand, attempting to sit up and stabilize his shaking legs. I tried to move the suitcase—packed the previous night with caregiver Joan's help—and nearly fell over. It weighed a ton and was bursting at the seams. I unzipped it and found it filled with files and books, but no clothes. There was no room for them.

"Can I remove some of the books? You won't need them all, like this one by Trudeau." I proceeded to put the book back on his desk.

"NO!" Bobby tried to stop me and fell over backward, hurting his already swollen elbow.

Three hundred and forty days had passed since Day Zero. Bobby had spent the last four months at home, doing rehab as an outpatient at CGH. A constellation of problems had emerged with his coordination, movement and EQ—all from the untreated status epilepticus[17]. Nevertheless, Bobby was persistent. He wanted to pursue his ambition of becoming a neurologist, a lifelong dream that remained unshakable. Although his medical knowledge had returned at an early stage in his recovery, he was far from fully recovered.

Lately, Bobby had been attending the Friday neuro grand rounds at CGH. All the neurologists in the city would congregate to discuss critical cases. Bobby would go in elated, as if he were taking part in the discussions. Snippets of shoptalk occasionally wheeled home. "Your EEG was always normal; your case should have been discussed openly in grand rounds." You would wonder why Sand was so morbidly negative, someone had said. Some, however, from the feedback Bobby had gathered, didn't want a former patient to get the inside information. To them, Bobby was a living reminder of the perceived appalling treatment he'd received; to others, he was an embarrassment. He attended the rounds anyway.

Bobby sat on the edge of his bed to put on his socks. Normally, he looped his left arm around the Saskipole, leaving both hands free for the socks. Not this time. As he lifted his shaking right foot, he fell forward onto the floor, face first. His glasses gashed his left eyebrow, barely missing the eye. He couldn't move; he just remained on the floor bleeding. Until I could get him up, I didn't know the extent of the damage. I was scared. A sense of despair and hopelessness descended upon me as I cleaned the blood off his face. The wound wasn't deep, and the blood quickly stopped rolling down into his eyes, but his glasses were all crooked. Relieved, I lay down beside him, thinking and praying. Two accidents in a row on the day of departure. God, help me. How am I going to pull this off?

I had tried to talk him out of going back to Montreal, and into concentrating on his rehab, but he wouldn't budge. An occupational therapist at the CGH had convinced him that he wouldn't improve anymore, and that he should go back to Montreal, because "the hospital won't provide active treatment for life." He'd had several interviews in Calgary, with Dr. Antel, who'd visited the Health Sciences Centre, and with Dr. Smith and others at the med school. He had written four abstracts for the ensuing Neuro conference, all of which were accepted. Finally, in early May, he had received the letter from Dr. Francis, offering him conditional acceptance as a resident at the MNI. But Bobby needed a full time attendant to take up the offer. He had only so much energy; if he used up most of it in caring for himself, none would be left for his career pursuit.

PART 4: MONTREAL, 1995

The doorbell rang and Joan appeared. She was calm and strong, a battle-hardy fifty. She took Bobby by the arms and gave him a good bath. He refused to have a shave; he'd packed away the shaving kit in his suitcase. The cabbie came a good half hour early and waited patiently while Bobby downed his bran and raisin as Gale took video; she hadn't done this the last time. Neilly took off to school without saying goodbye, and Mon went to her work at the hospital. The neighbor's son came by and offered to mow the lawn, trim the hedge and spray dandelions. I hadn't had time to look after the house or its other inhabitants.

Bobby snored through the flight to Montreal, and snored away the night in the apartment hotel, while I struggled to keep up with his medicine schedule, personal care and food. He could doze off at any time and in any place. When he did, which was often, he would break into a thunderous inhalation–exhalation sequence of "Grr . . . rr . . . rr . . . fss . . . ss . . . ss . . . grr . . ." Once in a while, he would hold his breath for what seemed like an eternity before letting out "fss . . . ss . . . ss . . . ." To wake him up in the morning to the point where he could swallow ten of the thirty pills he needed each day was a task of mammoth proportion. My wobbly job situation wouldn't let me remain in Montreal for long. I had been nurse, patient advocate, porter and travel agent. I'd become a peanut activist as well, writing letters to Hollis Harris, then president of Air Canada, to lobby against serving peanuts on the flights. But I would have to return to Calgary. I needed to find my replacement within the week.

JUNE 5, 1995. IT WAS A RUSH DRIVE TO THE MNI, where Dr. Antel was holding an early morning session with his residents. The meeting was already in progress, and Bobby joined in, behind the closed door. For me, it was a victory of sorts. I had wheeled him back from the jaws of death to the residency program of his choice. I celebrated the momentous occasion with a filming spree in the empty halls of the renowned institution. No one to witness but the video camera, and no one to share with but the spirit of Dr. Penfield[18] and his message in the display case: "No man alone."

MEDICAL MALADY

Reality set in in a hurry. I needed to put the finishing touches on the support network I had set up for Bobby, the network that would allow him to survive and function in Montreal. Before long, it was time to pick him up from the MNI and return to the hotel.

On the drive back, Bobby revealed more about his out-of-body experience while in the coma. He had started to tell me about it in bits earlier, but we had never finished the conversation. He'd found himself walking in a cave with a little girl holding a teddy bear, toward a bright yet serene light. As they got closer, occasional sparks flew. Suddenly, the girl stopped, turned to him, and said, "You have to go back, Bobby. If you or any of your friends get a cat, call it MYNX." She vanished into the brilliant light and Bobby found his body in a morgue, covered in a white sheet. His coma dreams began to unfold from there in twenty-two episodes, like a box within a box, twenty-two times. He could see his past, present and future lives as he got out of the boxes, one at a time. The episodes were as complicated as they were protracted, and they had begun to fragment and fade from his memory. His walk in the cave, however, remained crystal clear. I dropped him off at the hotel and went to the JGH.

By the time I returned in the evening—following a fleeting appointment I had made with Dr. Scho in the hope of getting some answers about what had transpired—Bobby had a handful of visitors: Liette, the OT from CLSC[19]-Metro outreach; Louis, from Lifeline; and Ian St. John, about Bobby's age, from the McGill University office of students with disabilities. Assistance with daily living, emergency response and homecare were in place, but transportation remained unresolved. La Tour was out of range for McGill's handicap bus, and Medicar and STCUM[20] were unreliable for early morning appointments. The homecare attendant offered to help with calling taxis and assist with transfers.

Bobby would use a Lifeline panic button that he'd wear around his neck. In an emergency, someone would respond through the speaker within the guaranteed sixty seconds and call the police, ambulance or a hierarchy of responders. That included the apartment hotel manager, Bobby's friend Barry and myself. He wouldn't have to reach for

PART 4: MONTREAL, 1995

the telephone to answer calls, as the Lifeline equipment had a two-way speaker with added functions. We hoped this would make it possible for him to avoid falls.

JUNE 7. IT WAS MY LAST NIGHT OF CHAPERONING. I heard a plea, "Can you help me go to the bathroom?" Bobby had forgotten to take his puffer. He sounded a bit wheezy.

"Sorry, I won't be here tomorrow. I have to watch you help yourself so I know you can manage on your own."

Bobby stood up from his bed and waited until his myoclonus subsided to steady himself. He then transferred himself to the wheelchair. Repeated training had paid off. For a normal person, the move would be automatic, but for Bobby at this stage of recovery, every step had to be executed consciously every time, or the consequence would be severe.

Ian appeared at 6:30 A.M., clean-shaven and cheerful like the rays of sunshine that needed no "hello" or "good morning." It was all over his face, the way Bobby used to be before his injuries. He would return in the afternoon, at 4:00 pm, to take charge of Bobby's personal care. I had given the CLSC a printed copy of Bobby's allergies and care needs and handed one to Ian as well. "I will miss you, Dad," Bobby said, as we parted. It was a rare display of emotion.

BACK AT LPH, THE COMA DREAMS are dispersed and dissipated, like clear blue sky at the height of winter. Bobby has found himself confined in this icy oasis, his mind fractured by years of adverse counseling. If he could only rid himself of the suspicion drilled into him by the lawyers, he would realize that his family is not his enemy. The real enemy appeared as a friend, and then left him in the wilderness and vanished with his settlement money.

I want to know everything that happened in those years—what he was told, what he did. But before he will reveal what happened to him when he was cut off from his family, Bobby wants to know the rest of his story.

21

REJECTION

DECEMBER 1, 1995. IT HAD BEEN SIX MONTHS since I'd left Bobby in Montreal in the care of Ian St. John and the CLSC. My work had mostly been in the east, making it possible for me to visit him often, bringing the medicine and supplies that Gale would pack for him. I could buy groceries so he wouldn't starve, I could check for any physical catastrophe that had befallen him and needed attention, and I could also help widen his network of support. This time, however, it was different. I left Calgary, worked in Florham Park, New Jersey, for the week, and flew from Newark to Montreal. The plan was to help him get to his LSAT exam at McGill on Saturday, a back-up plan, and then take him back to Calgary with me on Sunday. The night before, Gale had mentioned the name Alfonso, which hadn't rung a bell, so I called on arrival at Dorval, something I wasn't in the habit of doing.

"Do you have some food? Has Alfonso cooked for both you and me?" I asked.

The CLSC had replaced Ian with Eric, whom Alfonso had, in turn, replaced. Eric, a New Brunswicker who wanted to be a nurse, was not only a trained homecare worker, but also an excellent chef. He was young and doughy, much like Bobby had become. If Eric had been there, I knew I'd get something to eat.

"Mm-hmm," Bobby replied, enigmatic.

"Do you want me to do some shopping for you?"

"Sure."

"What do you like? No, what do you absolutely need tonight?"

PART 4: MONTREAL, 1995

He rattled off a long list: one tomato, one cheese stick, one pepper; it went on and on. Then he added, "three cans of pop and one package of toilet paper—no, no, lots of them." He didn't have toilet paper. This had happened last time, too.

"How ya managing, crusty bum?" I poked, to lighten the situation. But he seemed lost in thoughts of his predicament.

We had moved Bobby from La Tour to Peel Plaza during Neilly's summer holidays, a year after Day Zero. Neilly was furious. "This vacation sucks; you are spending way too much time here with Bobby." He was ready to rebel when I felt a sudden twitch in my lower back, just as I was about to cart boxes from the elevator. He pushed me aside to rest and heed the early warning sign and volunteered to move the boxes to the apartment. "If you die, then what?"

On the day Bobby signed the lease agreement with Peel Plaza, Dr. Francis told him that he would need a quantum physical improvement before he could handle neurology. Bobby wasn't ready to accept this news, and he didn't want to leave Montreal. Impulsiveness took him to Victoria, B.C., to attend the Canadian Congress of Neurological Sciences and present papers that he had authored and co-authored. But what he needed most was more physiotherapy, not research papers. On his return from the grueling week away, he couldn't function as well as he thought he would.

Yet Dr. Antel kept him on the payroll and gave him plenty of notice to get further rehab and find a less onerous program that would suit his needs and aspirations. On that premise, he bought basic furniture for his apartment on credit, and asked Gale to bring a long list of household items—bed sheets, pillows, toaster, plates, pots and pans, cutlery, his favorite childhood items and, of course, more books— with which, whew, we complied and crammed into the cramped La Tour before moving him to the spacious Peel Plaza.

Starving, I entered the apartment. The airport exit had become a maze; missing one exit took me to a spaghetti jungle, and backtracking in the dark had taken the last hour.

Bobby ate leftover rice and veggies, plain and simple. No food for me; the fridge was empty. I opened the cupboard to look for something to cook for myself. Out came a deluge of dirty dishtowels.

"Any clean towels?"

"Nope."

"Why doesn't Alfonso keep the dirty towels where they belong?"

"The closet is full."

"Is Alfonso coming to do the laundry tomorrow?"

"No, today was his last day until I come back."

Come back? Not likely. Not to the MNI, I thought, although I knew Bobby liked Montreal. They treated him as a colleague, not some patient. But they had ordered neuropsych tests, his second time since the coma. Memories of the leading questions asked at FHH—on family dynamics—lingered in our minds. This time, however, there was no hidden agenda. The MNI wanted to test Bobby's capability in carrying out his duties, in addition to his physical functioning. Dr. Aubé—the neurologist—was concerned about his attention span. I wasn't a bit surprised; keeping Aubé's appointment had been arduous—a nine-block manual wheelchair ride, enough to drain away anyone's focus.

Dr. Leonard, the neuropsychologist, said that, fundamentally, Bobby had two deficits: physical and neuropsychological. Anyone could see his physical deficits. The neuropsych evaluation, however, needed careful analysis. Drugs and drug interactions can certainly affect neuropsych test scores, but drugs didn't explain his deficits entirely. Leonard wanted Bobby to go back to Calgary and concentrate on his recovery—on such things as computer skills, typing, and analyzing current events. Being in Montreal would hinder, not help, in getting back to the practice of medicine.

A few days earlier, Eric, with whom Bobby kept in touch, had taken Bobby to a Lebanese restaurant. Bobby suffered a seizure, perhaps a mild one. No injuries, and the little sac of fluid on his right-elbow was getting smaller, but it was still red. Since then, however, he had been completely wheelchair bound, less steady on his feet. Even transferring seemed difficult. But when Dr. Aubé said, "Bobby will recover

PART 4: MONTREAL, 1995

more; there's still room," he seemed happier to remain in Montreal and sort out his options. There was a fair amount of scatter in his neuropsych test results, showing that his injuries were responsible for his neuropsych deficits.

"Why is the dishwasher full of dirty dishes? They smell," I asked, frustrated.

"Alfonso doesn't know how to start the dishwasher. He hasn't been in Canada long."

I thought I had one job; now I had three: cooking, laundry and the dishes. I needed to clean the bathroom before I could use it and wipe the mud and wheelchair tracks off the living room floor so I could unroll my sleeping bag.

I began the grunt work with the dishwasher on the fifteenth floor, and the laundry in the basement. Up the sloth elevator back to fifteen, I started preparing a salad and a sandwich. Bobby watched and swallowed his saliva. He hadn't had much to eat.

"Do you want some?"

"Sure." He devoured half of my sandwich in one bite.

I went down and up many more times to check the dryer, but the clothes stubbornly remained wet to the touch. After an hour I brought them upstairs, semi-dry, and went to bed exhausted.

Sleep in this apartment was as foreign to me as the appliances were to Alfonso. If it wasn't the flashing neon lights on my face through the curtainless sliding balcony door, it was the thermostat that didn't modulate with the temperature setting. Hot water would gurgle through the heater pipe or not come at all. I got up to turn it off when the room became too hot to bear, and to turn it on when I nearly froze. The thin blanket and a sweater weren't enough to keep my carcass warm on the floor. Bobby snored away bare-bodied, matching the rumble of the dishwasher, the blue comforter on the futon in his bedroom unused beside him. The blubber that protected him from freezing moved with a sudden jerk of his diaphragm and tapered off as he exhaled.

The alarm blared, uninterrupted. I got up an hour late, in a near panic. We had to be at McConnell building by 8:00 A.M. or the scribe—a PhD student in psychology—would leave.

The LSAT exam was a protest, an act of frustration following a series of failed attempts in quantum physical improvement. The signs of these failures were all around the apartment. The gypsum wallboards in the living room were decorated with gouges, dents and cave-ins. The bedroom wasn't spared. There were gouges on the wall at the far end. Bobby remained dependent on the wheelchair. There was no shortage of neurologists, epileptologists, neuropsychologists, and neuro-critical-care specialists at the MNI—a bonus of being in the nerve center of neurology—and Bobby had seen them all. There were neuro-rehab facilities reasonably close as well. He tried electromyography and physiotherapy sessions. The results were the same: no fast cure. He attempted to reduce his medications to improve his attention span, with devastating consequences in terms of seizures. Edith, a twenty-five-year veteran physio-rehab therapist at the Royal Victoria Hospital, spelled it out for him. "It's too early for you to get back to work, Bobby; you should go back to Calgary and recover." She went on. "You don't listen to me now, but you will when you find yourself in bed or in the toilet for two days."

His dreams of being a neurologist taken away, Bobby tried a residency in psychiatry, a close relative that didn't demand physical dexterity. I went with him to see the psych secretary–coordinator for the residency program, an enchanting, plump redhead with a large dangling nose ring. She was bright, talked through her lips, hands, eyes—in fact, her whole body—and set up five interviews in a jiffy with her wit and charm.

Two days later, we waited for an hour for the locked gate of the Allen Institute of Psychiatry to open, and nearly gave up. It was a Friday, during summer holidays, and there was no one in sight. Suddenly, someone appeared, quietly opened the lock and vanished without saying "hello" or responding to our "thank you." Bobby peddled through Room 101, the stable—the name carried over from the past, when patients used to be transported by horse-drawn wagons—to Room 103 for an interview with the chairman.

PART 4: MONTREAL, 1995

The meetings and interviews went on for months. Finally, the psych panel determined that the rigors of residency would be onerous at this stage of recovery, even for psychiatry, and encouraged him to reapply in six months. The Quebec referendum arrived in time to distract Bobby from his predicament. He ignored the terse letter from the Department of Psychiatry and embraced sick leave. As an alternative, he chose to write the LSAT.

But we needed to get there first. Sixty centimeters (nearly 2 feet) of wet snow had fallen in Montreal on December 1, 1995, turning existing mounds of snow into ice and slush. Conveniently, the city cleaning crews went on strike. Bobby asked me to park the car in front of the gate and wheel him in. I could barely grip the ground myself; to push the wheelchair with Bobby's weight on it was impossible. We were nearly twenty minutes late. We found the scribe pacing the floor nervously, contemplating a day's pay vanishing in the snow.

It was a different world, flying Bobby back to Calgary on a commercial flight. At Dorval, I parked his wheelchair in the Maple Leaf Lounge and ran upstairs to get a hamburger for his on-board meal—Air Canada couldn't guarantee the peanut-free meal that A&W could. On the flight, Bobby settled in his seat next to me, deep in sleep. His roaring snore attracted curious looks from fellow passengers, some laughing to hear him that loud. The bothered look on others' faces wasn't a bother for me. He was safe.

22

EVIDENCE

JANUARY 12, 2003. ABOUT TO SWALLOW A CHAMBER-FULL of pills from his weekly dosette, Bobby stops and smiles. "You're obsessed," he says. "You remember it all." A relaxed tone, given the predicament.

"What they did to you changed all our lives," I say, sighing. "Left the wound raw in all of us, or I wouldn't care."

Gale knees the refrigerator closed, peeks into the dosette—Neurontin and Lipidil capsules, along with other medications—and hands him the bottled water we picked up on our way back from Hoito's, a Finnish eatery in Thunder Bay.

"I could go on, if you like."

"Please, go on," he says. Exuding the politeness of a freshly minted psychiatrist, Bobby swallows his pills in one gulp. It's as therapeutic for him to listen as it is for me to recount.

JANUARY 18, 1995. I SAT ALONE ON A SHINY LEATHER SOFA in the claustrophobic waiting room, surrounded by a heavy wooden door, a receptionist's desk, and the frosted wall of the glass office facing me on the 31st floor of the Canada Trust Tower. Below the frost line, I could see a pair of leather shoes, crossed. The shoes shuffled, the roller chair moved, and a heavy-set balding man came out through the left side door. He ushered me into his plush chamber, complete with a floor-to-ceiling skyline—my first visit to a lawyer's office in Calgary.

Brian—a middle-aged, mild-mannered medical malpractice lawyer with a background in criminal law—started to turn the pages of the

PART 4: MONTREAL, 1995

document I'd dropped on his executive-style desk. It wasn't the principles of justice that brought me in, it was the desire to decode the death warrant. I needed to know what had happened to Bobby on Day Zero.

Away from the clutches of the hospital social worker, and returning to Montreal against all odds, Bobby had finally realized that his untreated status epilepticus had destroyed his fine motor control, making it impossible for him to pursue his dream of becoming a neurologist. As devastating as this was, it made it easier for me to deal with his next question. "I'm trying to get back to the medical profession—how can I sue them?" Doctors, physiotherapists and friends in Montreal convinced him that it would be okay to sue the specialists, even though he was trying to become one. Jen, too, needed to be in the mix. How else would the truth be found about what had happened that night?

Brian stopped short of the last page: "The Statement of Claim must be filed at the court within one year of injury." I'd heard that from Doreen, a lawyer in Edmonton. The one-year rule—the statute of limitation period—seemed designed by the doctors for the doctors. It's a dreadfully small window. Fresh out of a coma, Bobby was unable to focus on anything but the activities of daily living and recovery during that time. He didn't know what a lawsuit was, much less how to launch one. For Gale and me—carrying on a demanding full-time job, maintaining a family with two other children, caring for our disabled son, dealing with the detractors—life was busy as it was. A lawsuit was onerous, but time didn't have to be against us as well.

A preliminary investigation was needed to determine the merit of the case. That required the opinion of a medical expert on the standard of care, as well as an analysis of medical records, literature and case law. It would take a month, perhaps more, depending on Brian's schedule and the schedule of his expert—if he could find one to take on the task. I placed a limit on his involvement—around the Calgary hospital only—to keep the cost manageable and protect our rights in Alberta. The statute of limitation in Quebec was more humane: three years. We'd loop them in later.

MEDICAL MALADY

Trauma had robbed Bobby's memory of anything that would implicate Jen, but Brian's background in criminal law led him to question her assertion of the Chinese take-out. He wondered "whether there really was a take-out at all, or, whether in fact Bobby had eaten at the restaurant." It was a question that was consistent with our own observations. If she could be made to testify, we might finally get at the truth.

Those "ifs" were hurdles that hinged on finding not merely a medical expert, but one who would stick his or her neck out to support the case. Brian wanted an intensivist—a high-priced ICU doctor—to begin with; Doreen, the lawyer I'd consulted in Edmonton, had suggested a neurologist.

Dr. Mukherjee could shed light on the rationale behind the withdrawal of anticonvulsants in the ICU. He didn't see eye to eye with Dr. Sand, although Sand was one of his students. Close to retirement, he would perhaps be willing to talk.

He was—at a secluded Earl's Restaurant on 4th and 24th. Sand and Lee had "quietly tried to say goodbye to Bobby." He did not know why. He had "stepped in and told them that it's too soon. International code called for 30 days, and no withdrawal of medication." The damage had taken place on the very delicate cerebellum—affecting speech, balance and eye focus. His advice was to get the medical records—right away, or they might be doctored or, worse, disappear. There were two recourses: legal and political. He couldn't be our expert. We needed to find someone who'd had nothing to do with Bobby's treatment.

I wheeled Bobby to the Medical Records office in the basement of FHH—shortly before he left for Montreal—and deposited $300. The documents arrived in a few days, five hundred pages of loose leaf photocopied papers in a packet. I punched holes and organized them with tabs. Mukherjee had been right. Brian's summary noted, "There is curious note by Dr. Fox on page 49 which has been scratched out…" But the records were largely intact; they weren't electronic, thank goodness. Those files can vanish with the click of a keystroke.

Doctors "doctoring" documents, I said to myself. I'd be damned.

PART 4: MONTREAL, 1995

The JGH records had yet to be retrieved. I knew a bit better this time to ask for not only the medical records, but for emergency treatments, emergency doctors' and nurses' reports and notes, ICU doctors' orders and reports, nurses' notes and reports, laboratory reports, neurologists' reports, reports on EEG and CT scans and notes of all consults. They responded: "First twenty pages are free but there is a charge of $0.25 per page."

The pregnant medical records—another nearly five hundred pages—were delivered, and I took them to Brian. The X-ray films and EEG tracings that I hadn't asked for soon became crucial.

Shock and awe lurked in the first few pages: glaring gaps in the ER record, a pen that had overwritten the time of arrival had—or appeared to have—written a false neuro-consult report, citing "cardiopulmonary arrest lasting ~5 to 7 minutes"; false information elevated Jen's status in the JGH ICU, stating that Bobby had been "living with his girlfriend, a medical resident as well."

Medical records weren't sacrosanct in this domain of distrust, where rights, truth and values—even when life depended on them—could be trampled.

A corporate lawyer colleague at work had mentioned the name Gordon, a noteworthy malpractice lawyer in Montreal. I went and left a binder containing the JGH medical records with Gordon on my solo visit to his office. But it was necessary to bring the target of the misery with me.

Bobby's wheelchair felt heavier as I pushed it from the underground parking puzzle of One Place Ville Marie to Gordon's vintage office. A personal injury lawyer for twenty-five years, with a claim to fame of three wins out of four—a high batting average, perhaps from careful screening; three separate cases this month alone—pointed to many major malpractices in Montreal. Damage in the black box of the brain? It would be easier to prove if the head was chopped off by mistake!

Gordon was gruff and graphic. He announced that not one of the players in his network of medical contacts was useful in coming up with the goods, except to say that the doctors and the hospitals involved were big guns, not small fry in a teensy clinic. With Gordon's focus on quick wins, the case would be too complicated and time consuming; he had only so much time and energy.

I was shunted off to Jean-Pierre, a fee-based lawyer, close to my work in Montreal East. It took twenty minutes to get to his modest office on a non-descript street between Notre Dame and Sherbrooke, past the Olympic Stadium. A tall, polite, heavyset man in his fifties, he listened for a short time, and then handed me a bunch of documents written in French, outlining the terms. The only page in English was the one that described the Fee Agreement. Like most lawyers, a retainer paid in advance opened the door to a dialogue.

I took a detour around to Gordon's office on the return drive. He had made up his mind; it was too difficult a case: the girl wouldn't cooperate, doctors would hide information, the burden of proof would be on us. But, he reiterated, that didn't mean we didn't have a case.

JUNE 30, 1995. DAYS FROM THE DEADLINE, a year from Day Zero, Brian filed a $4.4 million lawsuit in the Court of Queens Bench of Alberta, against FHH and a handful of Calgary ICU doctors. The Statement of Claim (SOC) wasn't immediately served. The case against JGH and the Montreal doctors would have to wait until we resolved jurisdictional issues. We wanted to keep the costs to a minimum, and to channel our resources to Bobby's recovery and his career. A *Calgary Herald* reporter got wind of the lawsuit through a routine examination of the daily court filings and published an article[21], shattering any hope of keeping the matter quiet.

Hell and fury broke loose. Calls kept coming—to the lawyer's office and to our home. Bobby started to shake when I told him about the newspaper leak. The occupational therapist was upset. The CRHA team of healthcare professionals that worked with Bobby following his injury—to keep the lawsuit at bay—was dismayed.

Dr. Mukherjee was fuming. He was named in the lawsuit, despite having saved Bobby's life. But leaving him out would have provided an escape route for all the offending doctors, Brian had advised. Gupta

PART 4: MONTREAL, 1995

and his wife were furious as well: they had brought in Mukherjee. We became social outcasts, the target of harassment at social gatherings. The telephone stopped ringing.

The newspaper didn't know to report that Brian wanted out. His efforts had produced no credible medical witness to support the case against FHH. Without one, there wasn't a lawsuit—just futile fumes and fury.

Brian had asked the opinion of an Edmonton ICU chief. Three months later, he sent in a four-page report by fax, a predictable dissertation of "exemplary" rhetoric from within the brotherhood of provincial teaching hospitals. Among others we approached was a neuropathologist from "Sand's backyard," and we went in never-ending circles with him. He was afraid for his job. We learned a valuable lesson: seek out-of-province witnesses or risk gathering useless patronizing medical reports, and bills.

"SERIOUS BREACH OF CARE and protocol," muttered Beatrice—an alert, personable figure in her forties—in a mix of French-Canadian English and gestures, as she filled me in on her findings. I had dropped in, on my way back to Dorval, from my work at the Montreal East refinery. She had been an ICU/ER nurse and metamorphosed into a malpractice lawyer in Jean-Pierre's law firm. Gordon had sent over the JGH records. Perhaps because of her background, I had the feeling she would be the one to keep digging. No one become comatose without cause.

The ER and ICU charts clearly showed Bobby's hypoxia wasn't caused by anaphylaxis, aspiration or cardiac arrest, as I had been told at JGH and at FHH; it was a foreign object that had throttled him and robbed his breath for more than an hour. The neuro consult report—"cardiopulmonary arrest lasting 5–7 min"—was one humdinger of a lie, a cover-up. Beatrice said she would consult with an anesthesiologist to comment on the case, and keep the cost down.

I was flying in anger—and vindication that I hadn't been wrong—as I left her office to face the murderous Metropolitan Boulevard traffic.

MEDICAL MALADY

I got to the airport in the blaring company of Radio-Canada, called Bobby from the Air Canada lounge to let him know that Beatrice uncovered the evidence we had been looking for, and boarded the plane for Calgary. Pilots and airlines couldn't get away with the kind of botch-up that had nearly dissected Bobby into a bucket of organs and left him disabled for life—why should the doctors and hospitals?

23

LOOP

DECEMBER 23, 1995. OUR OAKFERN HOUSE WAS ABUZZ with the cacophony of kids grown up, celebrating a very special birthday. Nearly everyone was from the Western Canada High, International Baccalaureate (IB) class of '89. Bubbly, blue-eyed Cheryl—Bobby's first debate partner at Western, the surprise guest of the evening—arrived from California without her saxophone, but made noises just the same. No caroling like the years before the coma, nor cake or candles, for safety's sake, but they all sang "Happy Birthday" spontaneously, reflecting a genuine love and concern.

Nearly all members of the IB class of '89 had done well in their lives; they had become professionals. Bobby, born with exceptional intelligence, was one of them—though he was now derailed, disabled and struggling to get back on track. It mattered little in this moment; the house was full. Bobby had returned to recover and rebuild his life. Mon and Neilly were at home, just the way they had been in Christmases past.

It was the tail end of the CaRMS match for a new crop of doctors competing for next year's residency positions. Bobby became involved in helping with researching medical witnesses, and kept in contact with McGill. Word of the lawsuit had spread in the Montreal medical community. "Bobby's case is well known," a neuro-critical care doctor on the fifth floor of the MNI surgical unit said. "What one learns as an insider is quite different from medical records." We met him in

Montreal. Bobby asked, "Is there a case against JGH?" His response was, "A good lawyer should be able to build one." He understood how the teaching hospital worked, read between the lines, and said so without hesitation. He would write up a summary as a friend, but a "forensic assessment" was a different matter. He couldn't be a witness. He would send the medical records to Annette, a lawyer known to him. Her husband was an ICU specialist at the Royal Victoria Hospital.

McGill told Bobby to go out of Quebec to pursue his career. It wasn't an unexpected repercussion. He started sending out papers for a CaRMS match in psych/rehab medicine and preparing abstracts for the upcoming neuro conference—all in Ontario. He got better at using the home computer, sent out and received faxes and typed up letters, slowly if he didn't have help.

WITH THE STATUTE OF LIMITATION criteria met, we gained time, but not much. It wouldn't be long before the Statement of Claim had to be served. Progress depended on a credible medical witness, but every medical witness in Canada not only belonged to the fraternity of doctors, but also worked for the same medical system that was to be sued to get at the truth.

I learned that a lawyer's hours are as impossible to track as they are inordinately expensive. An ordinary wage earner needed to seek a contingency arrangement, or risk heading for the poorhouse. But no lawyer would take a case on contingency without a medical witness, complete with balls big enough to testify despite the risk of being fired. It was a vicious loop. Naively, I forked out retainer fees—from my solitary paycheck—in different cities. After running around in circles, there was still not a drop of progress to show.

The path of a complaint to the medical associations and colleges regulating physicians wasn't straightforward either. They circle through never-ending committees leading nowhere. Incompetent pathologists, gynecologists, radiologists and other "logists" go on *ill-*practicing for years—without reprimand or redress, protected within the fortress of this self-regulating fraternity, until the damage is too

PART 4: MONTREAL, 1995

large to contain and the tsunami of public opinion overwhelms them. The reprimands that follow often seem a travesty.

Beatrice gave me reasons to move forward, to force the hospitals and doctors responsible to own up and admit to the truth she unearthed. On November 15, 1995, I took the day off work and went through the medical records. I plotted Bobby's oxygen partial pressure pO_2 and oxygen saturation O_2 *sat* from the blood gas analysis for the first few hours after his arrival at the Montreal hospital on Day Zero. The numbers took a plunge for over an hour and didn't fully recover for more than two. The correlation was irrefutable. Something had throttled Bobby, and robbed his breath for the duration.

Armed with graph, charts and a PowerPoint presentation, I headed for a meeting in a Nosehill neighborhood north of Calgary. The new information rekindled Brian's skittish interest. He wanted the wildcard neuropathologist from Sand's backyard to be present at the meeting. The neuropathologist wanted the meeting to be held in his mansion—in his boardroom-size kitchen, in fact. For four hours, we remained stuck in the quicksand of causation, unable to progress beyond the reasonable doubt of the devil's advocate. Exasperated, Brian said he would take the case on contingency if there were support from a neurologist. The wildcard suggested a neuro prof from Pittsburgh. Brian found a neuro prof from Hamilton, who had testified for the plaintiff against a little known clinic in Niagara Falls. He forwarded the medical records to both.

A month later, Brian received a terse twenty-one-line report from Hamilton—no charge, no support, and no surprise. The Pittsburgh report was tied up in knots on technical matters, and its author refused to take a position. I met Brian in his office and tried to impress upon him that the chosen witnesses were heads of neurology at medical schools, and therefore part of the system. They had little interest in finding fault in their own backyard. Brian wasn't convinced. I asked him to keep the file until I could find a solution.

On the way out, I passed the receptionist, yanked on the wooden door, and came face to face with a battered old apparition—the real reason why Brian refused to take the case on contingency. The woman was pushing the door from the outside to get in, just as I was about to go out. She stumbled in. I held the door open until she disappeared into the office. The receptionist whispered: "That's her." It was Dorothy Joudrie, the celebrity socialite who'd pumped six bullets into Earl, her oil-tycoon husband. Earl wanted out of their relationship. One of the newspapers reported, "Dorothy was deeply upset and in denial about her husband's decision to leave her." She'd called 911 to help Earl, but was nevertheless charged for attempted murder. If Earl was anaphylactic, I thought to myself as the door closed behind me, Dorothy wouldn't have needed a gun; she'd go scot-free.

O'Brien, a senior partner in the law firm, was deeply involved in the Joudrie case and didn't want involvement in ours, someone in the law firm pointed out. Brian's role, as he described, will not be "to continue on as counsel in a situation where the Statement of Claim must be served in the next few months, prior to the date of filing expiring." The chicken-and-egg loop of lawyer and medical witness was a tough shell to crack.

24

NETWORK

JANUARY 8, 1996. NIGHT CREPT IN EARLY in wintery northwest Calgary. Gale tugged closer and whispered, "You think we will find what we are looking for?"

I said, "Of course, it's a med school library after all."

We soon found ourselves settling down at a desk on the second floor of the Bach Centre, Mon's literature search neatly organized in a white D-ring binder beside us. I turned to the article on Lance-Adams Syndrome—brought on by hypoxic injuries—to look up the names of the authors, and then asked the curious attendant hovering nearby for The Official 1995 ABMS Directory of Board Certified Medical Specialists. Only a handful of Canadian neurologists were listed—not good. The Canadian Medical Directory for 1995 wasn't useful either; a number of neurologist names showed up, but with no coordinates.

A break came a few days later. A membership directory of the American Academy of Neurology for 1996 arrived in the mail, opening the door to a host of neurologists worldwide, and with it, access to the NeuroNet website. Bobby had applied for membership in the American Academy of Neurology. The timing was impeccable. We could pick and choose names from the directory and correlate them to our literature search. Gale and I made many more nightly trips to the med school library. The aim was to keep away from the big names in the literature—they were part of the establishment—and concentrate on the employees.

MEDICAL MALADY

THE LETTER-WRITING CAMPAIGN that followed worked. A respectable flow of email responses began to arrive, one sent on Tuesday, January 23, 1996, at 3:01 P.M.:

> "Thank you for sending me your well-prepared material. You have legitimate concerns. I have some difficulties with this, as I personally know some of the physicians involved. It would be hard for me to be totally objective. Alternative Canadian neurologists who would be suitable include: Dr. W.T. Blume, London, Ontario; Dr. R.S. McLachlan, London, Ontario; Dr. Allan Guberman, Ottawa, Ontario. American neurologists include: Dr. Michael Aminoff, San Francisco, and Dr. Eelco Wijdicks at the Mayo Clinic in Rochester, Michigan. I am sorry to not be of more help, but it is better that I bow out earlier than later."

A follow-up as well, sent Tuesday, February 6, 1996, 7:43 P.M.:

> "Apologies for the delay in responding to your email of Feb 2. I have discussed the issue with Drs. Blume and McLachlan here. Both feel very awkward, since they know one of the doctors very well. However, we collectively came up with the following names of very suitable Canadian neurologists who should be at "arm's length" from the individuals involved. These are: Dr. David MacDonald in Vancouver; Dr. John Wherrett, Toronto; Dr. Donald Paty, Vancouver; Dr. Trevor Gray, Toronto; Dr. David House, Kingston; Dr. T. Jock Murray, Halifax; and Dr. William Pryse-Phillips, St. John's, Newfoundland. I think you will find any of these individuals to be very suitable."

Suitable, maybe, but a collection of the unwilling. I would soon learn why. The search for a witness geared up to the next level.

25

MATCH

MARCH 6, 1996, 2:30 P.M. THE TELEPHONE RANG AT WORK. I sensed it was Bobby. I wasn't sure why he'd be calling; I'd just spent the lunch hour with him at the Eau Claire Y following my daily workout and stayed to watch him swim. Linda, the swim instructor, took him from the warm wading pool, with adjustable floor, to the colder, larger pool designed for length swimming. He enjoyed the supervised therapy and attempted to show off his lost swimming skills (from Bronze Cross and Bronze Medallion programs), despite my ongoing worry that another disaster might lie in wait. In the disciplined environment of home, he hadn't had any major incident (or seizure) since moving back from Montreal. I often wondered what the Sow had had in mind, trying so hard to remove him from home.

Bobby kept a busy recovery schedule, complemented with drug treatment. Using Handibus for the disabled to get around, he exercised with a volunteer on machines at the Y, had acupuncture and music-therapy with alternative-therapy specialists, visited CGH physio and the one that tilted the ground—that psychologist, the Psy. The activities helped him cope, regardless, and kept him on an even keel physically, despite his disabilities. I was able to leave Oakfern even for a week-long business trip to France. Gale, however, remained under pressure in dealing with the demands of the disabled, as well as Neilly's various activities. She derived strength from Mon's excelling in med school.

"I am matched somewhere," an exuberant Bobby announced.

"Where?" I asked.

"I don't know yet, but somewhere."

Somewhere would have to be in a city in Ontario, a neutral province in his matter; and it'd have to be either Ottawa or Toronto. He'd secured interviews for psychiatry residency positions at the Royal Ottawa Hospital of Psychiatry and at the Clarke Institute of Psychiatry, Toronto. With no time to recover from the jetlag on my return from France, we were on our way to Ottawa first, and then Toronto. Before his injuries, I'd accompanied him to Toronto for his interview in neurology. From there, he'd gone on by himself to Ottawa, so full of life, hope. This time however, he needed help—big time.

In Toronto, I wheeled Bobby to the interview room on the eighth floor and left the building through the College Street exit to walk around the neighborhood for exercise. Then I gravitated to the Clarke cafeteria with my "office"—the laptop. No interruption here, just the usual goings-on, with one exception. Outside the door, a disheveled, spirited man in tattered clothes was lecturing to an invisible audience. I couldn't hear him, but I wondered, what had driven him to this madness?

Lunch for Bobby was guaranteed peanut free. Unlike in Ottawa, I didn't need to run lunch from McDonald's to the interview room, and Bobby didn't need to puff Beclofort or pop pills to stabilize his stubborn myoclonus. He emerged triumphant in Toronto, following the two-hour interview over lunch that had stretched to five hours. The opportunity gave me time to work on the contact that an old classmate of mine in Ottawa had given: a San Francisco neurologist with Canadian experience.

WHEN I FINALLY DID GET IN TOUCH, THE NEUROLOGIST gave me and earful on mismanagement in the Canadian healthcare system—health insurance funded by the taxpayers. "Standard of care costs no more money to deliver, and yet a lack of checks and balances makes it unavailable to Canadian patients," he said. "A case like Bobby's would never happen in the U.S., despite all the adverse propaganda. Discontinuing anticonvulsants while patient was seizing...!" and "government regulates treatment

PART 4: MONTREAL, 1995

in Canada…principles are not in writing; it would be an embarrassment if they were," and "the case would be a very strong one in the U.S., but in Canada the doctors are essentially employed by the government, protected by the government," and "the organization being sued is being witnessed by the same organization." His message was clear: our quest for truth behind the curtain of "internal hanky-panky" would be no less traumatic than the injuries that had necessitated it.

26

FLASH BACK

APRIL 29, 1996. MONTREAL AGAIN. Gale donated her Air Canada companion ticket so that Bobby could accompany me to Montreal, and a month later to Toronto. Peace of mind was more important to her than a complimentary trip around the world. We hadn't had a vacation together since his injuries.

For Bobby, Montreal was unfinished business. I drove him from Dorval to the apartment he retained on Peel. A mere five months before, excitement and myoclonus would've taken control of his hands, feet, parts of his face and indeed his entire body as he'd unzip the pouch around his growing waist to take the keys out and attempt to find the right one to insert into the keyhole. His hands would bounce up and down, refusing to cooperate. His face and toes would twitch as his hands would finally settle, but only his thumb and index finger would go to work. The rest would remain idle. Since then, he had made progress and his movements attenuated, but they were far from gone away. His stopover here was to look for neuro advice and support from his Montreal mentors.

I took Bobby to Kathleen—a neuro-physiotherapist at L'Esprit Sports medicine centre (and a PhD candidate in Rehabilitation Science, McGill University)—and watched her as she demonstrated the effect of his injuries with a plastic volleyball. "During the coma," she explained, "he [Bobby] went into status epilepticus, and it took several days for the brain seizures to be appropriately controlled." She continued, "The neuronal damage has resulted in a constellation

PART 4: MONTREAL, 1995

of problems in his coordination of movement. These coordination problems affect both movements at a fine level as well as movements involving the whole body."

His next stop would be Collin, one of the neurologists at the MNI, who'd motivated him to write down his memory flashes—it would be therapeutic, he'd said. I wouldn't be there for that meeting; I'd have to leave to catch a flight.

Leaving Bobby to his own devices wasn't as distressing as it used to be, knowing he was in good hands. Ian—whom Bobby had called to help during this month-long stay in Montreal before moving to Toronto to start his residency training in psychiatry—was both dependable and punctual. He would look after him, morning and evening. Grocery shopping and cleaning that I'd done would last through the month when I'd return to shift him to Toronto. And yet, it was painful to picture Bobby in a wheelchair in downtown Montreal, or any inner city for that matter, at the mercy of passersby to get him across large intersections when Ian wasn't around. On occasion, Bobby had seized uncontrollably, leaving blood and skin on the sidewalks, and scrapes or fractures on his face and extremities, attracting onlookers until someone would call for help.

CLEVELAND. THE LAST TIME I WAS HERE ON BUSINESS, I'd used my spare time to look for a cure for Bobby's injuries. This time, however, I was looking for a medical witness—a neurologist, to be precise. In a stroke of luck, I found one listed in the Elyria-Lorain area, not far from my work. I made an appointment at the end of the day and drove to East River Street, knowing little of what the cost might be, or whether I'd end up being thrown out of the office. I was prepared either way, following encounters with several imposing doctors. One, an anesthesiologist, had appeared difficult when I'd met him in the presence of the fee-based lawyer, Jean-Pierre. But when I met him on my own a few months later, in his tastefully decorated condominium in Ultramont, he appeared normal. He heard our story patiently and became quite emotional. He talked openly about the poor treatment his first wife had received in a Montreal hospital before her passing, and about his three kids, all of whom were from his first marriage, and all allergic. We became friends in a very short time and before I left, he made a prophetic remark in line with the comment that the San Fransisco neurologist had made, that came to be partly true as time progressed: A negative aggregate of perpetual penury.

This Cleveland neurologist was acutely aware of his own situation. A nondescript doctor in a nondescript small town in Ohio, he was brutally frank.

"Look, to be honest with you, it's not worthwhile for me to testify, leaving my practice here. Besides, I am a neurologist of Indian origin; they may hold that against Bobby."

"I understand," I said as I viewed the wall of certificates behind him.

"If you have to have a hired gun, your best bet is to get one of the biggest ones who really understand hypoxic encephalopathy."

"How do I know who does, without wasting a lot of time?"

"I would give you the names I know; others advertise in legal magazines and journals."

He contemplated for a minute or two and recited at ease: "Fred Plum, Jerome Posner, John Hughes, Victor Maurice," and gave me a brief background of each. I left an hour later, no charge.

The visit kicked off another letter campaign—this one for potential medical witnesses in the U.S. The Cleveland list snowballed to cover leading authorities in the field, and the responses followed—like the one from St. Elizabeth's Medical Center of Boston:

> "Thank you for your letter regarding Bobby. It is quite a travail. If the details you recount are correct, then indeed things went very badly.
>
> I find myself in an awkward position of wishing to be helpful, but being completely overwhelmed with work of various nature at the moment. Furthermore, I have made it a strict habit not to participate in medical/legal matters because of the inordinate

PART 4: MONTREAL, 1995

amount of time involved. For this reason, I have had to decline getting involved in cases such as yours that have merit. I would like to help, however, by giving you the names of several colleagues who are experts in neurological intensive care.

With regard to the status epilepticus, I would certainly ask Dr. Ken Jordan, who is in La Jolla, California, or Dr. Thomas Belck in Charlottesville, Virginia. Also, Dr. Victor Maurice, a prominent American neurologist and the co-author of a major textbook, from time to time will testify in such cases. He is a Canadian and may have some disposition toward committing time to Bobby's case. He is currently located at the White River Junction Veteran's Administration Hospital in White River Junction, Vermont.

I wish you luck and I hope this has been helpful.

Sincerely,

Allan H. Ropper, M.D."

The letter produced a nugget, a shortlist, and the name "Jordan" proved to be one of the most valuable of all potential witnesses.

MAY 27, 1996. FLYING BACK TO MONTREAL, my mind was unsettled. I was anxious to see Bobby, not knowing what shape he would be in after his latest "accident." I hadn't seen him since I'd left him there, in late April, although we'd talked many times. Mon—on a break from her rigid schedule preparing for the United States Medical Licensing Examination—was on the flight too, her first trip ever to Montreal. I was eager to show her the ground zero of Bobby's poisoning and the disasters that followed, though I knew she wouldn't understand or feel the pain of a parent. The only other person who would was tied up with Neilly's Grade Nine provincial tests.

The door was open and the TV blaring the Stanley Cup hockey finals as we walked in. Sitting at the desk facing the wall, amid a pile of papers and a barely visible laptop, was Bobby. He was gulping every movement of the puck with the attention of a grown-up child, oblivious to the conspicuous cut on his left eyelid. The lacerations over his left temple spoke louder than the broadcast; it was a miracle that his left eye had been spared. Myriad facial cuts at various stages of healing left battle scars of seizures on his overstretched skin. His disheveled appearance—face full of beard, long hair and nails—matched that of an aggressive hockey player. Dust balls, wheelchair tracks and shoe marks covered the floor, while dirty dishes, stains and matted hair covered the countertop, sink and bathtub. His diet had deteriorated to scraping the bottom of a jam jar, and yet he'd gained a few pounds. He was out of breath. The only progress seemed to be on his paper and posters for the upcoming neuro conference. Also, he'd written a story about his coma dreams. More pointedly, he'd typed his memory flashes into his computer, one myoclonic keystroke at a time:

> *While his back is turned, Freda takes some peanuts from her pocket, chews them up and swigs the last of her glass of wine.*
> *Mark finds the glasses. "Excellent."*
> *Freda is startled and knocks over her wine glass. She turns around. "Great!"*
> *Mark starts to pour two glasses of port; he gives one to Freda and takes one for himself.*
> *Freda leans over and gives him a deep kiss.*
> *Mark smiles and downs the port in one swig. His face suddenly turns gravely concerned from its previous joviality. "There's something wrong with the port."*
> *"What do you mean? I tasted it—nothing wrong with it," says Freda, not even having tasted the port. "Why don't you try the rest of my port?"*
> *Mark starts to drink Freda's port. "No, it's not the port. Something else." Then he puts the port down and collapses.*

PART 5:
TORONTO, 1996

27

TRAP

APRIL 22, 1996, CALGARY. "Everything we do is on contingency," an affable male voice announced. It sounded too good to be true, but needed exploring. I scooted over for a face-to-face meeting. The office was tucked away in a corner of the fifteenth floor of the Home Oil Tower, a short walking distance from mine. Nearly all of the law offices on our list were within walking distance—a plus for a city where bubble-bridgewalks join buildings in the downtown core. A narrow entrance by the elevator banks led to the greeter, Jamie, a recent graduate from law school. His face held a gravity that made him look older than his age. It was a big office space for a two-man show, but they seemed hungry for business. An appointment with the principal lawyer was set for the next day.

"Fuck, it's an interesting case," Bill exclaimed. "I don't usually get much documentation, but there's no shortage here!" I'd brought a hard copy of my PowerPoint slides and my diary, and I went over our progress to date. I'd given the same presentation to many lawyers and medical experts of short and restless attention spans. It got easier each time.

Bill, crop-topped and balding, broke into a high-pitch braying laughter, making me wonder if he was right for the job. He'd just settled a case for million and a half with Brian as co-counsel, he said, trying to gain my confidence. He appeared enthusiastic, alert, quick on his feet. He spoke little but absorbed a great deal, much like Jim—to whom Brian's secretary had just sent the files, and whom I was also considering seriously. Bill was younger, in his early forties,

PART 5: TORONTO, 1996

and less inhibited. Unlike the others, he was willing to sue all parties, including the "princess" in the center who had apparently pulled the trigger that started the domino of destruction—a compelling point when it came to getting at the truth. His concern, however, wasn't the truth but a quick win, meaning settlement and compensation. The deal was struck with the understanding that if the case settled, our expenses would be paid, and if a felony was unearthed, files would be forwarded to law enforcement.

A trustworthy lawyer was an oxymoron to Gale. She'd refused to visit any of them. "Go ahead if it doesn't cost us any more," she would say, knowing well that injuries had turned an admirable asset into an enduring liability, and our savings were vanishing fast. I played it down. "It would be on contingency," I said, not exactly knowing what that meant. I had no experience in civil litigation, least of all against so many powerful and supposedly cunning defendants.

I'd asked for Bobby's Handibus to drop him off at the Home Oil Tower when he finished swimming at the Y. Bill was fast on his feet with the papers—as if he'd been waiting—the moment Bobby wheeled in. He had him sign the Contingency Fee Agreement, Patient Information Release and a number of blank pieces of printer paper; no date on any of them. Time was of the essence, he said. It was the week of Bobby's departure for Toronto via Montreal. Word of the lawsuit had gotten around.

28

ELM STREET

TORONTO, MAY 31, 1996. I WHEELED BOBBY INTO THE Mount Sinai Hospital residence on Elm Street early in the afternoon, long after our midmorning arrival at Lester B. Pearson airport. The traffic wasn't gridlocked, but there were airport delays, routine for the disabled. We had to wait for the wheelchair to come up from the cargo hold, which can happen only after all the passengers leave the aircraft. We could live with that and joke about it, but the challenge of finding a parking spot in the hospital district was no laughing matter. The parkade around the corner opposite the hospital had no in-and-out privileges and charged nearly as much as the daily rental car, well beyond the means of someone on a single paycheck with a brain-injured son. I double-parked on the street, to run up and drop off the luggage we'd brought from Montreal, and saw the movers had been in. Then I rushed off to the Bellwoods Outreach handicap services: homecare had to be arranged or I couldn't return to Calgary.

It seemed like a happy union when Bobby was finally introduced to his apartment on the tenth floor. However, he was dog-tired. And so was I, just looking at the scattering of unpacked boxes, furniture in wrong places, and his impulsive collection of swords, paintings, pictures, CDs and videotapes, all of which had taken him deeper into debt. He had a comeback. "They gave me a deal, ½% over prime!" His emphasis was on the ½%, not on the prime. The bank hadn't hesitated to give him credit; he was a medical resident, and in time might become a specialist, disabilities notwithstanding.

PART 5: TORONTO, 1996

Bobby couldn't keep his eyes open following our McDonald's lunch. I fetched his telephone, on a mission to find a private homecare service for the week before social services kicked in. The Spectrum agency found Kesh, an athletic, laconic homecare man in khaki and bright new running shoes, who showed up at 5:00 P.M. on the dot. A new immigrant, with a master's degree in economics from south India, he was unfamiliar with the system and unsure of how to deal with a peanut allergy, so uncommon in his vegetarian world. He needed training in caring for a brain-injured man with extreme sensitivity to nuts, and I needed help with the apartment and installing handicapped fixtures. The building superintendent and the maintenance man advised that we find an outside contractor. It was just as well that Bobby was deep in sleep while the man of economics got trained—and the kitchen and the rest of the apartment got fixed—or he would have played down his disabilities in a feat of overconfidence and assured Kesh that he could do everything himself. But when fatigued, which was often, he would forego the basic elements of daily living and live in the detriment of doing without.

The apartment began to transform itself into a livable space for the disabled. I'd visited it when it was being prepared, during one of my business travels, to check out the handicapped access through another building—I had them remove the doors between the rooms for wheelchair movement—and to meet Fay, the congenial, middle-aged building superintendent who showed me around. The building appeared older than Peel Plaza. The bedroom and living–dining rooms were joined through an elongated kitchen at one end and the hallway entrance and bathroom at the other.

There was no hardwood floor here, just tightly laid off-color office carpet, giving off the sweet smell of bug spray and exhibiting ubiquitous roach traps. No roaches could possibly exist here without gasping for breath, I thought, and welcomed myself to the Toronto apartment scene. Fay played it down. "We spray and keep traps as a preventive measure; besides, the tenth floor is hard for roaches to climb up to." The proximity to Mt. Sinai—where Bobby would be first assigned—

was a blessing and made it worth putting up with the roaches. For access to his place of work, he would go down the elevator to the basement, negotiate a ramp into a long and desolate underground utility tunnel, and surface in the basement of the hospital across Murray Street. He needn't venture out on wintry nights when the weather might bring freezing rain. The downside to the tunnel was the absence of a support rail on the ramp, and the desolation. But the ramp was wide enough, and Bobby was recovered enough to counter both, or so I thought.

Dinnertime rolled in as I pushed the weighty wheelchair down Dundas in search of a Swiss Chalet; we had no groceries yet. The flat terrain of Toronto seemed safer than Montreal for the manual wheelchair. Amenities and conveniences were within easy wheeling distance: place of work, banks, Hasty Market, even a gas station for pumping up wheelchair tires that went flat after a month of hauling expanding Bobby-weight. The streetcar tracks, however, were notorious for catching thin tires.

The following day, the task of carrying groceries from the parkade to the high-rise was grossly underestimated. This wasn't like Calgary at all, where Bobby used to help, carrying bags from the car to the kitchen, only steps away through the door between the garage and the house. The grocery store at DuPont and Christie was different, built in a festive style we hadn't seen before. It greeted shoppers with appealing ethnic food: sautéed spicy eggplant, green pepper and cauliflower cooked right there at the entrance on large hot plates. Served in a carnival atmosphere, complete with the sounds of songbirds and friendly people, the foods were without lists of ingredients. Bobby passed them in silence and then took full advantage of the rest of the store, buying much more than he could possibly use. He pushed the shopping cart ahead of his wheelchair like the choo-choo train of his childhood.

But after climbing the steep stairs to the building entrance, using one set of keys to open the door for each trip—up the slowest elevator since the JGH ICU—and then using another set to open the apartment, I finally rested on my aching behind. The final trip from the car

PART 5: TORONTO, 1996

park, with Bobby in the wheelchair, through handicap access at the other end of Elm on McCall in a different building, took two sets of elevator rides: one going down a floor to the basement, and the other—far down the basement hallway into another building—up 10 floors.

The elevator door opened with a clank. Bobby turned his head up to find a lanky brunette with a sad face carrying a laundry basket on her hip, as if she were carrying a baby. She cut her line-of-sight in half and held the door open as Bobby was about to use his legs to steer the wheelchair out of the elevator belly. Moments passed without a word, and then suddenly she asked: "How did you get here?"

Bobby recognized Krista, one of the Peccaries, now a second-year psychiatry resident at the Clarke. She lived in the adjoining building, with shared facilities. She hadn't the slightest idea that he was back on track in Toronto.

29

OFF COURSE

MAY 2, 1996. AN URGENT CALL from Jamie to say that they had received the files from Brian, the lawyer who'd filed the $4.4 million lawsuit at the Court of Queens Bench of Alberta on our behalf before dropping out. Bill, the new lawyer, was literally flying with the case—on his way to California. I had a hunch he was shopping for medical witnesses before he'd had time to review the files. That would cost money, and lead nowhere. My hunch was correct. Jamie gave me a draft report of the assessment written by a neurologist—at the Department of Neurology, University of California, Davis Medical Center—hired through Medical Expert Testimony. The doc missed the whole point, took the false neuro-consult report of five to seven minutes of cardiorespiratory arrest as a given, disqualified himself at the outset—"An assessment of the adequacy of his management during the first few hours of hospitalization is outside my area of expertise"— and collected his fees: 4 hours at US$350 per hour.

Prompted by the assessment, Bill asked me to drop JGH ICU and FHH ICU from the statement of claim: "Whatever happened to Bobby happened in JGH ER." I couldn't go along. The series of adverse events had started with Jen and ended with the FHH ICU. We couldn't afford to drop any one of the defendants. There were too many witnesses to discover, and Bill's failed attempt to find a medical witness played into his proposition. Upon studying the records, however, he confirmed that the JGH ICU neuro-consult report was false. We had known that the ER docs couldn't find Bobby's pulse for

PART 5: TORONTO, 1996

two to three minutes; they had noted it in their observation in the ER report. Someone got hold of that information in the ICU and blew it out of proportion: "cardiopulmonary arrest lasting 5–7 minutes." Drs. Koh and Leslie's notes appeared to have been replaced with the false report. It had caused irreparable harm in the course of Bobby's treatment, nearly terminating his life, and now it was distracting potential medical witnesses, sending them off course.

So when Bill made demands on us to dig for information—X-rays, EEG and EKG tracings, list of nurses and doctors, all my correspondences, diary and chronology of events, previous medical history and records, JGH telephone book, director of the numbered company that had owned the Chinese restaurant, their insurance company—we obliged, though it meant Gale and me working on Sunday—Mother's Day—or any other day that mattered or didn't. We delivered anything we found to his home, or to his office, in person.

Ironically, Bobby's return to Montreal's MNI was crucial in securing his CT scans, twenty-seven large X-ray plates, and two small ones that held the key evidence. He could read the small plates and discover the demon that had sat in his chest on Day Zero and mercilessly drained his life away, one frantic breath at a time.

30

LONDON

LONDON, ONTARIO. JUNE 26, 1996. The session was in progress. Quietly, I opened the door with one hand and pushed Bobby's wheelchair into the large auditorium with the other. Pitch dark it was, but I could sense the hall was filled to capacity, and all eyes were on the distant brilliant overhead screen, high above the stage. I parked Bobby by the projector at the back wall. Morning sun had followed us southwest, the day before, to this prosperous university town where, in the convention center, the 31st meeting of the Canadian Congress of Neurological Sciences was being held. We had checked into the Radisson next door on King Street. All four papers or posters that Bobby had authored or co-authored had been accepted. He would concentrate on presenting them, and I, registered as his companion, would help him. In between, I would scout for medical witnesses. I had missed the opportunity the year before, when the conference had been held in Victoria, and it had set us back a year.

My weeklong "holiday" had begun three days before, when I walked into Bobby's apartment. He was sitting on a rickety rosewood chair at his desk, which was stacked high with journals, books and his laptop, barely visible through the clutter of the coffee-stained papers, meds, and salt and pepper shakers. There was no room for eating or working. Disability kept him from filing things away. Instead, they piled up in one place or another, causing tripping hazards that resulted in conspicuous battle scars—on Bobby's knees, elbows and face. The Fibromyalgia-Myofascial paper was on display, and he appeared to

PART 5: TORONTO, 1996

be talking to Myosymmetry, the sponsor. Hearing me coming, he cupped his trembling hand over the ketchup-stained telephone and asked, "What should I charge, $50?"

To that, I replied, "Can he cover your out-of-pocket expenses?" I would look after mine—companion registration and two nights at a hotel. Though wobbly for walking and weak on financial dealings, Bobby could shave and dress on his own and do his packing, albeit slowly. He was ready early and eager for the session, but his knees hurt. He wanted to be pushed rather than to wheel himself in the morning.

Vision adjusted, I could clearly see the little man on the big stage focus his laser pointer on a key item on the screen that resonated with us both. His eloquent, authoritative voice propelled me to move closer to the dim light of the projector, rest my Hilroy notebook on Bobby's back, and start scribbling:

"Seizure identified early by EEG initiates early recovery without negative sequalae; chronic facial movement, twitches, chewing shows status epilepticus, diazepam ineffective cardio depressing, phenytoin (Dilantin) good, dose 18 mg/kg, EEG to monitor seizures, inadequate dose—seize, don't wait, add another 7 or 8 mg/kg, watch BP, respiration and hyperthermia (fever)."

He made it abundantly clear that seizures—convulsive, non-convulsive, burst suppression (the last of five stages of status epilepticus), myoclonic or whatever—must be aggressively treated. Seizures left untreated or poorly treated would cause brain damage by neuronal exhaustion.

If JGH in Montreal and FHH in Calgary had followed this simple advice, and the well-established treatment practice, Bobby would be writing his own notes, I thought. The speaker was Michael Aminoff of San Francisco, an advocate of proper management of seizures in the ICU.

A panel discussion—on electrophysiological studies in critical care units—followed. Near the end of the session, a humble voice from the middle of the now illuminated floor took command of the microphone and raised what I thought was a crucial point: "If a doctor prematurely diagnoses a coma patient PVS, the management of that patient becomes consistent with that diagnosis and the outcome becomes a self-fulfilling prophecy." It struck a common chord in layman's language—if the doctors say the patient won't live, the nurses stop caring and the patient stops responding.

The minutes until the end of that morning session seemed like an eternity. I rushed through the crowd of neurologists, epileptologists, psychiatrists, neurosurgeons, researchers and nurses to meet this humble saint of a man with a strong sense of social justice, leaving Bobby at the back wall. He was Dr. Seshia, a renowned neurologist and a specialist on coma. I introduced him to Bobby, and without hesitation, he became interested—a serendipitous break.

31

MOMENT OF PRIDE

SEPTEMBER 1996. IT HAD BEEN THREE MONTHS since Bobby had started his psych residency in Toronto. He had had three rotations modified to accommodate his disability in internal medicine. He said he might have saved at least one life, by admitting a TIA (transient ischemic attack) patient who was being sent home, perhaps to a full-blown stroke. It was a moment of pride for one whose own existence had nearly been terminated.

My work in the east often brought me back to Toronto, where I traded my hotel bed—two blocks down Elm Street—for one on the floor in Bobby's apartment, to help with activities that his new caregivers—Joseph, a stoic immigrant from Ghana; Darryl, a heavy-set humorous fireball from the Caribbean; and Ken, a despondent Toronto native, taking turns two hours daily—couldn't provide.

Saturday morning, I dropped Bobby off at the Mt. Sinai ER for his new rotation and went shopping at Kensington Market in pouring rain. Hours later, not quite dripping wet, I ventured into the restricted personnel area and asked for Bobby.

The nurse hesitated. "The doctor in . . ."

"Yes, the doctor in a wheelchair." I was in a rush.

"What's the problem?" The doctors and nurses in the area hurried in, in anxiety; they had reasons to. I didn't resemble a patient, nor a staff, but a storm-swept piece of driftwood.

"No problem; not at all," I said, trying to calm the situation.

That wasn't nearly enough. A bouncer of a volunteer popped up to usher me outside. Luckly, just then, Bobby sailed his wheelchair in on the polished floor, gleaming in a white lab coat with a Littmann stethoscope around his neck. "Hi, Dad." Anxiety vanished from the face of the doctors and nurses, as well as the volunteer. He took me into one of the consult rooms. A pleasing sight, and yet the doctor was in a wheelchair. He had to tell his patients that he had MS, just to shut them off, so he could concentrate on their afflictions, and not his.

I slipped a Timex Ironman wristwatch I'd bought on sale for $70 over Bobby's left hand, gave him a hug, and told him that the spare key I'd made for Krista, one of his classmates we had met, was on the dining room table, and the electric shaver was fixed and charging in his living room. The weather was turning uglier—hurricane Fran from the Gulf had started to be felt in Ontario—when I returned to the apartment, pumped up his exercise ball, cut a fruit platter for his snack, took the coral gold ring his grandma had given him for health to resize, left a note on his desk, picked up my laptop and luggage and headed for the car. Rain poured in through the windows that I'd left open in my rush, but fortunately, the wind was blowing from the passenger side. I was nearly dry as I headed for the airport.

32

SNOWBALL

TWO YEARS FROM DAY ZERO, an amended Statement of Claim that included both Alberta and Quebec doctors and healthcare facilities was filed for $20 million in the Court of Queens Bench of Alberta Judicial District of Calgary, with a notice to the defendants: *"You have been sued. You are the defendant. You have only 15 days to file and serve a Statement of Defense or a Demand of Notice. You or your lawyer must file your Statement of Defense or demand of Notice in the office of the Clerk of the Court of Queens Bench of Alberta."* There was an added warning: *"If you do not do both things within 15 days, you may automatically lose the lawsuit. The Plaintiff may get a Court Judgment against you if you do not file, or do not give a copy to the Plaintiff, or do either thing late."* The amendment strung the defendants from the Quebec and Alberta jurisdictions together—JGH and FHH hospitals; Montreal and Calgary doctors; Jen, the Chinese restaurant and defendants yet to be disclosed.

The support of the two principal experts—Jordan and Seshia—raised our confidence to serve the amended SOC. Support from two big-name experts snowballed as Bill and his secretaries—Chris and Marnie—worked through the list of experts I'd prepared. A personal campaign meant much more than a fly-by-night letter or a cold call from an unknown lawyer's secretary. At the London conference, Dr. Anderman, Bobby's neurologist in Montreal, advised me to deal with the lawyers, and the lawsuit, on my own, and keep Bobby away from it. His daughter was in the same psych residency program. There wasn't much choice but to adhere to the doctor's advice: medical residency was all-consuming, even for an able-bodied doctor. Other specialists in the conference privately provided encouragement to pursue the matter for the betterment of the profession, and in the interest of the patient population.

33

IMAGES

OCTOBER 1996. BOBBY'S NEUROLOGIST was on the other end of the phone. It had to be serious, I thought, for Dr. Gordon to be calling long distance. It was. Bystanders had found Bobby in a pool of blood that afternoon. His wheelchair had toppled as he was returning from work, and his forehead had hit the pavement at the corner of Elizabeth Street. They helped him get to the Mt. Sinai ER. His shakes weren't going away, although he'd stopped seizing. Gordon would increase the dose of Gabapentin he'd introduced after the second of the last three seizures in as many weeks.

The incident reminded me of a conversation I'd had with Bobby a few weeks earlier. "I won't have to do graveyard shift anymore," he said. "I need a volunteer scribe and they aren't always available; that slows down my ER work nearly to a halt." His program coordinator had arranged a family medicine clinic at the Woman's College Hospital, where Bobby evaluated twelve patients a day. It took an exhausting fifteen minutes of wheeling to get to work. Following the previous seizure, I'd met the neurologist, a plump personable man in his fifties whom Bobby revered as his surrogate father for ordering a motorized wheelchair to ease his travel stress. But the wheelchair had yet to arrive.

I located him after five telephone tries. He was on a stretcher in the ENT. The nurse appraised the devastation—his nose was swollen, seemed fractured. A couple of hours later, I could talk to him over the telephone. In a slurred, nasal whisper, he said he was being kept overnight for septal hemorrhage, a blood vessel rupture from the broken nose and a hairline skull fracture.

MEDICAL MALADY

The episode brought me back to Toronto in the middle of a general strike by Ontario labor unions against the Mike Harris government. By the time I left my luggage in his apartment to scoot over to Mt. Sinai, Bobby's childhood friend and his wife had already arrived. She narrated the scene and the sight—of lacerations on Bobby's bloody, battered face from uncontrollable rubbing on the pavement—that had made her feel faint on the night of the seizure. Bobby asked her to sit down, offered her a drink and said, "No point in us both getting sick."

I returned to the apartment at night, exhausted. The predicament had sapped my energy, even to turn on the lights. The dark blue curtains on the picture window—in the living room where I made my bed on the floor—allowed diffused city light, which made indiscernible images on the wall. The convective quiver of a large Canadian flag from the Quebec referendum campaign—hung from the curtain rod in Bobby's bedroom, seen through the narrow kitchen joining the rooms—was barely audible in the background. I knelt to lay down my head. A sharp shiver went through the nerve endings of my skin. Perhaps weakness took hold of my mind as well. I felt the presence of some energy form, maybe the same one that woke Bobby up from the abyss, watched over him and kept him alive for whatever purpose. It could have watched over him, a few days before, on the morning of the first of the three seizures, when Joe had fled the apartment, leaving Bobby alone with a grand mal seizure. The newcomer from Ghana had never seen anyone seize before, nor did he want to. Had the spirit also watched over him on the day when Bobby found himself on the floor, with a sore ribcage, sore nose, hurt knees and a memory gap of several hours? His wheelchair was kicked over, folded, collapsed off its moorings. Perhaps the energy prompted him to push the Lifeline button shortly after regaining consciousness and orientation, and alerted the paramedics and the responders. That very day, a letter from Edmonton awaited him in his mailbox: the University of Alberta had accepted him for law school—a tempting way out.

34

HOOK

JANUARY 9, 1997. A LETTER ARRIVED from Bennett Jones Verchere (BJV), acting on behalf of the CMPA—the doctors' malpractice insurer sponsored by the government to protect doctors against victims of medical malpractice. We hadn't heard much since the SOC was served, barring rumblings. "The parties are defending the lawsuit," the letter said; a Statement of Defense would follow. In other words, BJV was defending the doctors. Bill was hoping that a defense lawyer named Mart would be their lead counsel, for "he is good at what he does." It sounded strange coming from the plaintiff's lawyer. Other perplexities were popping up as well, all of which seemed more than a slew of coincidences.

A fraud investigator from the Alberta Family and Social Services called me at work. She wouldn't share the specifics, but she left the impression that Bobby was being investigated for fraud. Why she would be calling me, and not the social worker who had known his activities and whereabouts, was baffling. The CGH, which had provided a drug for free, to help Bobby walk better, demanded the money back. If that wasn't enough, Canada Revenue Agency nitpicked on his tax returns that I filed on his behalf.

Bill asked me to pick up the BJV letter from his office. He made it sound mundane. But nothing could have been further from the truth. I read the demands: school transcripts, IQ tests, income tax returns, receipt of prescriptions, early photographs, video as a young man prior to injury, clinical notes, paid care, EEG, on and on the list went. It seemed detractive—a make-work project—but its implications went far beyond simply making more and more money for the lawyers. The reason why Bobby had been in a coma was in the charts, and CMPA already had their hands on them. Besides, we had been told his discovery would be simple; after all, he had been in a coma. But the lawyers were adamant; they needed the information now!

There was one other puzzle in progress. The psychologist at FHH continued to provide psychoanalysis sessions whenever Bobby was in town (twenty-one times between December 1994 and May 1995, and seventeen between December 1995 and April 1996) and produced provocative reports: "His experience within the hospital and with his parents also contributed to his feeling infantilized and powerless. Upon returning home, he found himself having to deal with his parents' overprotectiveness and with others' attempts at protecting him from possible failure." "Therapy continued to address the themes explored in our previous course of treatment: the loss of Bob's fiancée; his feelings of alienation from his parents because of their rejection of her; the loss of most of his social support network; as well as the loss of physical functioning and its implication for Bob's personal and professional life."

I became interested in the "psychological treatments" the Psy had been providing, presumably to help Bobby, but perhaps also to help the employer—the defendant hospital. Bobby and I had met with her for an hour. She began referring to his brain injuries as "Bob's *mental* illness," indicating, "Bobby is doing it to himself by being careless," and, "Bob thinks you as parents would be hurt if he does not recover . . ." I wondered if she was rewriting history in a fragile mind—all his and his family's fault—and if we'd become unwitting helpers in a grand scheme outlined in some *legal* operating manual. CMPA, I gathered, was looking for a lawyer to act on behalf of the "girl" dubbed "Bob's fiancée."

35

CORNERSTONES

WEDNESDAY, MARCH 12, 1997, 9:07 A.M. THE CONFERENCE CALL was kicked off, a week late. Bill turned the speaker in my direction, across his desk, when Dr. Jordan came on line. We exchanged few pleasantries; time was of the essence. Bill briefly went over the expert's qualifications, and Jordan began to summarize his findings from his review of the charts that had been sent to him earlier in the year: "Bobby had an asthma-like response on that gruesome night, not sure if it was a full-blown anaphylactic reaction . . . he did not have a cardiovascular collapse; hypoxia only . . . when he was paralyzed, nobody knew what went on inside the black box of his head, neurologic evaluation had been meaningless, patient wouldn't respond, muscles paralyzed, eyes wouldn't open . . ." The hour-long exhaustive exchange was a preview to the upcoming discoveries and the expert reports.

With Jordan firmly on board, Bill asked me to see Dr. Seshia in Winnipeg over the weekend, on my way to Toronto. I was going to pick Bobby up from Toronto and take him to Montreal on Monday. With the medical opinions of Seshia and Jordan being the cornerstones of our case, I didn't hesitate to stop over in Winnipeg.

MARCH 14. THE CBC WEATHERMAN ANNOUNCED -25°C as I drove off in the rental car from the airport on my way to downtown Winnipeg. Silhouettes of scantily dressed teenagers appeared on street corners, puffing smoke that hung in the air. Aging automobiles moved lazily along the wide and open intersections, long trails of exhaust

MEDICAL MALADY

fumes in their wake. Early the next morning, I trudged over the snowbanks from the parking lot to the ground floor of the Harry Maclovy apartment building, near the Children's Hospital where Dr. Seshia maintained a modest office.

The electric kettle came to a boil as we exchanged small talk. No sooner was the tea ready than we got down to the business of the pointers Bill had asked for prior to the discovery. He'd sent over a thousand pages of charts, from JGH and FHH, signs of which were strewn across room 107. Seshia had pored over those pages with the thoroughness of a beaver.

Bobby was "alert and oriented" when he arrived at the JGH on June 30, 1994, Seshia pointed out; he was neurologically perfect. There was no notation of "Code 25" to indicate the need for resuscitation, nor any notation of "Code 99" to indicate cardiac arrest, and yet there it was in the chart: "Cardiopulmonary arrest lasting five to seven minutes."

"There are medical issues, ethical issues and social issues surrounding this case," Seshia went on, and he pointed to the pitiful state of the charts that no one addressed, no one had time for, and few appreciated. "The system failed Bobby," he said simply. "The system came out short in every department." I departed for the airport, satisfied with the support.

One solid support led to another as I buried myself in a report on the flight to Toronto, titled "Critical study of the medical record of Bobby . . .." It was written by a retired anesthesiologist—an associate professor of anesthesia at McGill University—and it focused only on the ER treatment at JGH. He had reviewed Bobby's medical history and charts with the utmost care and concluded, "Thus one can estimate that this adverse iatrogenic situation (high intragastric pressure, impaired diaphragm movement, presence of a foreign body in the bronchus) may have prevailed for two (2) full hours." Although he didn't mention the possibility of falsification of charts by the hospital staff—too polite and professional—that specter was raised.

Bill engaged a young and enthusiastic Quebec City lawyer, Marc, as co-counsel. The anesthesiologist happened to be his father. As honest as the report was, it provided only a valuable background.

36

BLOOD GAS

MARCH 16, 1997. BOBBY'S SOFT PALATE VIBRATED boisterously as the flight left Toronto, drowning out the noise of the takeoff—as if to announce to the world that he was coming to discover the truth, the whole truth, and that nothing could stop him from finding out. Notwithstanding the flight attendant's chuckle as polite passengers pretended to concentrate on the *Sunday Star*, the roar of his snore carried on until the plane landed in Montreal. By the time the wheelchair was brought up from the cargo hold, he was fully awake and we were the only ones left on the plane. The delay didn't matter much, as Bill's flight from Calgary wasn't scheduled to arrive for another hour. The wheelchair and all eight pieces of luggage—including Bill's file box, hauled from Calgary—loaded into the full-size red Taurus I rented from the National kiosk at Dorval. I began the milk run to Hotel Auberge, where we were to stay for the week, and to the Hotel du Parc, where Bill had rented a room for the night.

The next day was the first in our journey to hear the testimonies under oath. Bobby—still seizure prone, on thirty pills a day, and deep in debt—was pumped. Pushing his wheelchair first thing Monday morning—to McCarthy Tetrault on the fifth floor of the Bronfman Building at Stanley and Cyrus—was a cinch when he was wide awake and cooperating by paddling with his feet.

The atmosphere in the boardroom was businesslike, thick with anticipation. No more than measured pleasantries were exchanged between the plump, rosy-cheeked middle-age lawyers—one of them represented the CMPA for the doctors, the other for JGH—peering over the volumes of open medical charts on the rectangular table separating us. The proceedings were kicked off by the court reporter, Annagret Rinaldi, officiating at the head table. She was primed with equipment for transcribing every utterance for the public record. Towering behind her were two picture windows; on a tray on the sill was a large pitcher of water and several upsidedown glasses. Bobby was a silent observer, as was I on his right. I was ready to slide notes—to Bill, the plaintiff's lawyer on his left, or to Marc, the Quebec City lawyer next to Bill—on yellow 3M-stickies, to cover points overlooked, or to be alert and available to be consulted during the planned frequent breaks.

The sixty-six-year-old staff radiologist, now seated across from us and next to his lawyer, swore in at 9:00 A.M. Although I was drained—physically and financially—I recognized this man as if I had seen him before, for I had read his terse comment on the ER radiology report a thousand times. It didn't matter to me that my meager means were stretched to the limit; I'd stopped keeping track. Incredible as it seemed, our tax dollars were paying for the defense.

The credentials and credibility of the witness established, the process and timeline in the hospital clarified, Bill fired salvos read from his newly acquired laptop. Questions referred to the relevant pages of the records, choreographed with an agenda, as if he was taking macaques back to the murky waters of Mozambique, making them drink, over and over from various angles, until they spat out facts that rang true and clear, matching the malady. He danced around the crucial questions before asking them; he took impromptu detours, made adjustments, rephrased, restated and dodged objections kicked up by dozy opposition counsels, and kept the witness—well dressed and well prepped—on track, away from side-stepping or blaming the innocent.

Did Bobby have a "massive aspiration" on Day Zero, which is what we'd been told when we got there? Bill circled around the questions before getting to the point:

PART 5: TORONTO, 1996

Bill: With the improved density that was appearing on the third plate, did you assume that in fact there hadn't been a problem with aspirant in the lung or did you even address your mind to the issue of aspirant in the lung?

Rad: There probably wasn't. No, there was no indication of it.

Bill: Okay. And nobody asked you to look at the issue of aspirant in the lung. Is that right?

Rad: No.

Bill: And characteristically, an X-ray plate of the chest would show the presence of aspirant if it had been in the lung for a prolonged period of time, correct?

Rad: Yes, people can aspirate without anything going into the lung.

Bill: Right, but if they aspirate massively into their lungs, there will be—

Rad: You would see it.

Bill: You would see it.

Rad: Right.

Bill: But you didn't see any evidence of that.

Rad: No.

The morning went well, dispelling the myth of massive aspiration with ease. The infamous X-ray plates that had been taken following intubation hadn't been read by the radiology residents or the staff radiologist on call until the next day. There was no request to read the X-ray plates on a "stat" basis, the radiologist said, thus shifting the blame to the ER docs. One of them, thirty-seven-year-old Dr. Rose, appeared at 2:00 in the afternoon, following the lunch break.

The session was about to resume. The ER doc was on the hot seat when Bobby pulled out one of his dosettes, opened two chambers, jerked his stooped head back, way back, and emptied ten capsules and pills into his mouth. His meds were due. Someone with little knowledge of his myoclonus handed him a glass *full* of water from the jug on the sill. The glass shook, shivered and took a wrong turn to lay empty on the defense papers. Dr. Rose's deposition got off to a soggy start. The rush of paper towels sponged the moisture off the pages as we anxiously waited for the weary ER doc to pick one of the four options that dangled before him—take the blame, spread the blame, shift the blame or claim nobody was to blame.

Bill: Right. Were you the responsible physician?
Rose: I was one of the responsible physicians.
Bill: Who was the other?
Rose: Dr. Koh and Gra.
Bill: And doctor who?
Rose: Dr. Koh and Gra.

The option of spreading the blame appeared irresistible. But did he think that the cardiac arrest—that I had been told of—had been a myth? If not, Code 99 would have been called, and the ER doc would know the whereabouts of the code form that had recorded the event.

Bill: . . . you're telling me that a cardiac arrest can occur in the Emergency at . . . on June thirtieth (30th), nineteen ninety-four (1994), without anybody taking a minute-to-minute record of what occurs, drugs administered and who's there. Is that right?
Rose: I believe that the nurses record what was given.
Bill: And the best record that you say is generated in those kinds of circumstances is typified by what we see on page 13 of the documents.
Rose: He did not have a cardiac arrest.
Bill: Oh, he did not.

A forthright admission from the ER doc—who had been there and had taken part in the treatment—that Bobby hadn't suffered a cardiac arrest. There was more:

PART 5: TORONTO, 1996

Bill: So in this case we have no code sheet, correct?
Rose: Correct.
Bill: We have no attendance of the trauma team at the hospital. Is that right?
Rose: This was not a trauma.

Not a trauma, no massive aspiration, no cardiac arrest of five to seven minutes' duration—how had Bobby fallen into the cave of coma for twenty-four days? His stomach had been distended, pressure had been building up against his diaphragm, making it harder for him to breathe. His lungs had shrunk against such brute pressure. How? It made no sense. The day ended with more questions—a list of which I prepared—before dropping off Bobby and Bill at the front door of the Montreal Rotisserie Restaurant at du Parc. Snow made the entrance inaccessible by wheelchair from the parking area. Marc had joined in by the time I returned to the restaurant. The day's discovery suggested a total breakdown in the ER; everyone had been in charge, yet no one was. The dinner menu—a nut-free supper—preceded the next day's menu of doctors for discussions on strategy. Bobby was dismayed with the development, yet buoyed with the success of the first day. Truth had begun to emerge through the layers of lies, a little at a time. I slipped another list of questions to Bill.

THE NEXT MORNING, WE WERE BACK in the boardroom as Dr. Scho, the forty-three-year-old neurologist, sat on the hot seat. He volunteered on questioning that the book by Allan Ropper—with whom I'd corresponded, and who was distressed with the situation we'd encountered at the JGH—was the best definitive textbook on the treatment of convulsive patients. The discovery began in English at 9:31 A.M. Bill led the charge. The mission was to have the defendants own up to their mistakes, to link them to the vast array of damages. They had known their mistakes and had masked them with a neuromuscular paralytic agent, quoting such euphemisms as "movements" and "myoclonus" to describe the damaging symptoms of seizure. If the lawyers could demonstrate that there hadn't been any "seizure," then there couldn't be any damage resulting from it. The doc was allowed to play around with his version of events for the longest time, until the very end, when he was trumped to read—from his own handwritten notation on the charts—the dreaded words "status epilepticus" that he had avoided thus far:

Bill: Right, whether epilepsy or myoclonus, correct?

Scho: Well, and the initial insult that initiated it. You know, I have to clarify again that when you look at the ultimate— if you have an individual who is bleeding to death as a result of the fact that a limb has been hacked off, well, the damage has been done at the moment of contact of the axe with the limb. And what one does subsequently is to try to stop the haemorrhage, but the damage has already been done. In this particular case, the haemorrhage is indicative of the fact that the limb has been amputated. Similarly, in this case, myoclonic status epilepticus is indicative of the fact that there has been severe hypoxia.

Bill: So, what you are saying is that Bobby was such a case. In other words, his limb was chopped off by the hypoxic incident. And what followed afterwards was what followed afterwards, correct?

Scho: Correct.

Bill: So, can you show me the subsequent administration of the phenobarb?

Scho: Well, no, this is an order then to initiate and it continues. What I'm looking for now is an order to stop it.

Bill: Okay.

Scho: DC [discontinue] phenobarb on the order; that was on the 4th, so this is when I probably did it.

Bill: Okay, so, you cut it off then?

Scho: Yes.

Bill: And did you reinstitute it?

PART 5: TORONTO, 1996

Scho: Yes.
Bill: When was that?
Scho: So that the idea there would be to try and see what the clinical status was.
Bill: Right.
Scho: Phenobarbital was then loaded on the 5th, I believe.
Bill: Do we have the date shown on this record?
Scho: It is either 5 or 6. I can . . .
Bill: We can get to the clinical chart at that point.
Scho: There should be a notation by me. I believe that there should be—when that was initiated, there should be a notation by me as to the logic of that.
Bill: Sure.
Scho: Yes.
Bill: Where is that?
Scho: That's on page here, a little 57 on the bottom.
Bill: Okay, so 60 on your list.
Scho: It says he has, so this is on the 6th.
Bill: Alright.
Scho: It says: "Status epilepticus somewhat subject to realize tremulous jerking of jaw with rhythmic jerking of left toes and fingers." Right before, I note there is a Dilantin IV with fifty percent (50%) reduction in seizure. "Ativan formula abolished the seizure."
Bill: Yes.
Scho: "Will give phenobarbital five hundred (500) milligrams IV load."
Bill: Yes.

Bobby felt his arms, and the back of his head, and I felt a shiver as the lanky bearded fellow compared Bobby's hypoxic brain injury with the hacking off of a limb. Graphically, tenaciously, he elaborated the "moment of contact of the axe with the limb": "The haemorrhage is indicative of the fact that the limb has been amputated."

MEDICAL MALADY

The horror show couldn't end soon enough for me to seek relief. The rest of the crowd ventured out for lunch on their own, to return for the next round at 3:05 P.M. Bobby and I had a little conversation in a quiet booth of the restaurant, but contemplation of the hemorrhage was palpable—the seizure, the hemorrhage, the seizure, the hemorrhage, the seizure, the seizure, the seizure. It had hammered on Bobby, and our family, in myriad ways to this day.

Bill moved to Le Sanctuaire, Phase I, a tastefully furnished condominium belonging to the anesthetist's friend on Deacon. They were away. We met there for an evening strategy session for the big fishes the next day: Dr. DeM in the morning, and Dr. Spa in the afternoon. Bobby was drawn to the ornate chess set in the open concept living room. He invited Marc to play, while Bill pressured me for the electronic version of my diary. "There shouldn't be any secret between the client and the lawyer."

To that, I replied, "You have a hard copy already." He didn't have it with him; he wanted it for reference. I copied the version that Gale had typed up onto a floppy disk, showed him how to drag and drop the file from the floppy to his hard drive. He opened the file to verify. The game was over in six moves: Bobby had learned to checkmate a novice player, which the QC lawyer was. But he had to move the pieces for Bobby, who was gloating. "I am better brain-injured than you are."

Dr. DeM, 59, was on the witness chair on Wednesday. At issue was the integrity of the JGH charts. Bill attempted to suck out the internal reports of the treatment fiasco, but failed for all the objections. He took a different tack. The resident's consult report contained blood gas data that didn't exist in the lab printout included in the chart. The hospital produced the missing blood gas data through their lawyers, but it didn't have Bobby's name on it, and the time didn't coincide with Bobby's arrival, or the time of the claimed cardiopulmonary arrest.

Bill: As a result of the allegations of fraud in this case respecting the first blood gas result, what did you do in order to

PART 5: TORONTO, 1996

            retrieve the information that we now see contained on the two sheets of paper?
DeM: I went through the chart and the first two—that there was three blood gases comes on page 15 of the document, line 15, and that writes: "Investigation: . ."—I guess two points—". . . third ABG done."
Bill: Yes, and I had seen that as well.
DeM: And that bothered me. The second thing is I then wondered why there was a blood gas missing, and then in the admission—I couldn't understand the time recorded in the Emergency Room records on page 10 of the document.

A theme of disorientation and disappearance seemed to be emerging from the misharmony of medical care, and what seemed to be evolving—and I had been warned of it by the witnesses who wouldn't testify, a few who would, and those who were looped in—was a sheet music of broken trust. Would we ever find out the source of the malign melody?

37

DISCLOSURE

SPA MOVED FASTER THAN I'D EVER SEEN HIM MOVE. "Are you taking my picture?" he yelled. Positioning his massive body out of camera range, he summoned his lawyer, who was having conversations with other lawyers in the hallway. I'd put my video camera back into the case by then—I wasn't allowed to take pictures of the sessions, but no one had told me not to film at any other time. I'd taken Bobby into the boardroom ten minutes prior to Spa's examination, at 2:00 in the afternoon. He'd arrived early as well, and started talking down to the plaintiff in the wheelchair. I couldn't let the moment pass without recording.

The excitement settled, but, still coughing and wheezing, Spa sat down and took a couple of squirts from his puffer. His lawyer turned to Bill and quipped, "You wouldn't want to be in his territory."

Spa sniped, raising his head in a blink, "He will never get out." He didn't seem to be kidding, and his remark reminded me of the lawyer we had seen in his domain, tube-tied and horizontal, whose wife we'd had supper with in the hospital cafeteria in Montreal.

Elizabeth Robinson, the official court reporter, swore in Dr. Spa, 51. Bill began, in English. We'd heard in the earlier testimonies that "the intensive care is a closed unit. There isn't an order that is carried out without the consent of the physician running it." The physician on the witness chair admittedly ran the unit. He must have known what had gone on on Day Zero, and in the days following:

PART 5: TORONTO, 1996

Bill: Now, we talked briefly about the fact that Zan had mentioned to you the fact that there had been a misplaced nasogastric tube, which you thought was then functioning as a bronchial tube. Did you make anything of that in terms of the hypoxic episode that had been described to you?

Spa: No.

Bill: You just didn't consider that, or what?

Spa: The nasogastric tube, to my understanding, was placed in after the endotracheal tube, and the endotracheal tube was placed in because of the acute respiratory event.

Bill: Right, so you didn't think that the nasogastric tube was then going into the right bronchus, or what?

Spa: I mean, I was told that an X-ray was taken. The nasogastric tube was in the right bronchus and it was removed and placed into the stomach.

Bill: So you assume then that the nasogastric tube was not in the lung for any prolonged period of time?

Spa: My assumption was that it was in for a period of time from when it was placed in until it was removed, yes.

Bill: And did you then think of that in terms of the implications that that might have for a hypoxic patient?

Spa: Did I think of it? It certainly was not in the correct place; it should have been in the stomach.

Bill: Yes, well that is a slightly different question. I am just wondering, and I don't want you to go through a thinking process that you didn't go through back then, but to the extent that you can recall receiving that clinical information, as well as the fact that there had been a hypoxic event that had lasted approximately one hour as we saw in Dr. Cohe's [Year-1 resident's] consult note, did you think that the NG tube was implicated in that hypoxic event back then?

Spa: Did I think that—there was evidence of hypoxemia prior to the endotracheal intubation.

Bill: No, I am . . .

MEDICAL MALADY

Spa: And there was hypoxemia continuing following the intubation; a nasogastric tube was seen for a period of time in his bronchus.

Bill: Right, and did you link the two of them—the hypoxemia and the nasogastric tube in the lung—at that time, when you were told that information?

Spa: Did I link them to—?

Bill: In other words, you have a cavity, namely the lung, which is having oxygen pumped into it and an NG tube on suction. Did you link those two things and think, well, perhaps this is part of the hypoxia that Bobby suffered back then?

Spa: It certainly was a possibility.

For the first time, I heard Spa mention that the NG tube was misplaced in Bobby's lungs, and the tube was in suction, sucking oxygen from Bobby's lungs for a period of time. A reluctant admission to the falsehood we had been told in Montreal—that of massive aspiration—but an admission nonetheless extracted out of the veteran of lawsuits, with no objections thrown in by the defense counsel—spellbound in disbelief perhaps, or in a transient stupor. A bigger, more sinister picture seemed plausible: of the symbiotic relationship—of Spa and the two women befriending him with booze—following Day Zero and the push to keep us away, out of the scene, while they pretended to be the surrogate family.

AS THE DAYS OF DAMNING DISCOVERY progressed, the lawyers loosened and rumors of backroom offers flew. Jokes surfaced from the floor and bounced off the walls amid suppressed laughter. "Who pays the court reporter…?" "Big bill is coming to you…" "Alberta Heritage Fund pays…" etc. One remark compared the two-sided personality of the lawyers: primitive and refined. The sheepish witnesses came and went: the ER doc who couldn't or didn't read X-ray plates, a naïve R1 resident (Year-1 resident, also known as PGY1 resident) who wrote the

PART 5: TORONTO, 1996

falsehood as she was told, baffled nurses, an astute ICU fellow who'd discovered the near fatal iatrogen, and the staff docs who were left out of the loop. They all left their version of truth—truth that should have been told on our arrival in Montreal the day following Day Zero.

The nurse who'd treated Bobby in the ER said, "He was sitting straight up with his hands next to his body . . . he had been talking to us before. And then he sat straight up and he started saying, 'I can't breathe, I can't breathe, I can't breathe,' like that, and I just kind of had this chill. I just knew something terrible was going to happen." Just ahead of this point, a nasogastric tube—nearly five millimeters inside diameter—was introduced and connected to a wall suction line leading to a vacuum pump. Bobby became agitated, collapsed and lost consciousness. One of the ER docs had then intubated him, overlooking the misplacement of the NG tube. Another nurse who had come in following the 11 P.M. shift change said, "When I started my shift and I noticed it wasn't draining . . . so I did adjust it . . . the purpose is to drain the contents of the stomach. If the abdomen is distended and there is some gas there, they will come out . . ." But it wasn't the abdomen she was sucking the gas out of for the next nearly two hours; it was oxygen from Bobby's lungs. As he lay unconscious on the stretcher, no one knew or cared what was happening to him. Someone had called the ICU R1 resident, who'd called the ICU fellow, Dr. Zan, at her home. Her testimony summed it all up:

Bill: And when did you receive the call back to the hospital?
Zan: I'm not sure, but it's either a couple of minutes before midnight, midnight, or a couple of minutes after; it's all within that . . .
Bill: Okay, and do you recall who phoned you?
Zan: Yes, Cohe, the resident who was on that night in the ICU.
Bill: Okay. And do you recall whether or not a chest X-ray had been taken at the moment of your arrival?
Zan: The chest X-ray when I had finished my evaluation?
Bill: Yes.

Zan: I requested to look at the chest X-ray; it already had been done. So I don't know what time it had been done at.

Bill: Okay. Now, when you noticed that the abdomen was distended, did you make any investigation as to the cause of that?

Zan: Well, my examination took five to ten minutes to evaluate the patient, and just immediately after that I looked at the X-ray . . . I noted that the nasal gastric tube was sitting in the right main stem bronchus.

Bill: So, as soon as you saw the X-ray, you identified the problem with the . . .

Zan: And immediately asked, I mean, and the endotracheal tube was in good position. So immediately I asked that the NG tube be removed . . . I am unaware if I removed it myself . . . or if I delegated it, but it was done immediately after looking at the X-ray.

Bill: Okay. Now, the confusion that I have arises from the notes of Christine Egner [ICU nurse].

Zan: Okay.

Bill: Let's just take a look at them together.

Zan: What page are we looking at?

Bill: At page 15 in your record.

Zan: Yeah.

Bill: You'll see that on page 15, Egner writes a retrospective account of what happens at approximately 1:30 in the morning.

Zan: Uh-huh.

Bill: Do you recall reviewing the oximetry sheet that the respiratory tech prepared in terms of ongoing O_2 saturation as measured through . . .

Zan: At that time?

Bill: Yes, at that time or during that evening.

Zan: Reviewing it? No, I would—it was a visual—it was more visual.

PART 5: TORONTO, 1996

Bill: Okay.

Zan: I mean, looking at the oximeter in front of me.

Bill: Okay. Did the oximetry improve after the nasal gastric tube was taken out of the lung?

Zan: There was an improvement over the next twenty or thirty minutes or so.

Bill: Okay.

Zan: But the patient still, on transfer, was still receiving 100% oxygen.

Bill: Okay.

Zan: But the saturation was—on transfer—was up to about 90 or 94%.

No one had admitted to inserting the NG tube without checking its placement, without discovering whether it had ended up in the stomach or in the lung. Dr. Zan's notations in Bobby's charts disappeared like fugitive emissions from a toxic dump; you could smell them, but you couldn't see them. Instead, bullet points from Cohe—the naïve R1 resident—appeared as a neuro-consult report, to the surprise of one of the three ER docs:

Bill: Well, did you ever hear Gra or Rose ever tell Cohe or Zan when they arrived that evening that there had been a massive aspiration, a cardiac arrest lasting five (5) to seven (7) minutes?

Koh: I do not recall hearing that.

Bill: Did you ever talk to Cohe subsequent to the initiation of this suit or at any other time as to how she had come up with the information contained on her consult, which is page one twenty-four (124) of the chart?

Koh: I was not aware of this particular piece of information until the suit was brought forth, at which time I reviewed the chart.

Bill: And did you talk to her?

Koh:	I had not talked to her.
Bill:	So this is a complete mystery to you, is that right?
Koh:	It's a mystery in that we were the ones that were there; she was not.
Bill:	Right.
Koh:	And I would venture to say that our presence there, and Dr. Rose's note of two (2) to three (3) minutes is probably more accurate.
Bill:	Well, not only is it probably more accurate, it is accurate and this is false, correct?

Objection! The defense lawyer stepped in.

Koh had been present in the ER for the duration of Bobby's stay on Day Zero, before he was transferred over to the ICU. He could shine some light into the coma tunnel and illuminate the thinking behind the falsifying of charts, post event. No one admitted to a meeting on the botched ER work, a wall of objections was always thrown in the way. If the naïve R1 resident had been at that meeting, it would have been the perpetrators' last chance to instruct her to write the false neuro-consult report before she moved to her next residency rotation:

Bill:	Now, do you know whether the director or the morbidity committee have ever reviewed Bobby's case?
Koh:	This case was reviewed . . . In fact, we actually had a joint round with the intensive care unit that took place probably, you know, within a couple of months of the event, discussing the management of the case and how perhaps things . . . whether things could have been handled in a different way.
Bill:	And were you present at that meeting?
Koh:	Yes, I was.
Bill:	Can you tell me who else was present at that meeting?
Koh:	I believe Dr. Spa was there, myself, Dr. Rose, Dr. Gra,

PART 5: TORONTO, 1996

there were several other emergency attendings and ICU residents, and perhaps other ICU staff, but I won't specifically name them because I don't remember who was there.

Bill: Do you recall if Cohe was there?

Koh: I believe she was there at that discussion.

THE NAÏVE R1 RESIDENT HAD BEEN DUPED. She hadn't been qualified to write the lethal neuro-consult note. She had had little involvement with the case, while those who did wrote precious little. If they did write notes, as she testified, they'd have vanished, like the "yellow pieces of paper" she'd observed disappearing in the past.

Bill: Did you ever recognize that fact while you were treating Bobby? Did you recognize the cardiopulmonary arrest and the massive documented aspiration were in fact false statements?

Cohe: The aspiration now, only now I can look back at it, you know, but at the time, I don't know what I was thinking. At the time, I was just an Rl. Now I can, but now I'm looking back as an R4. It's different, you know.

Bill: So did Zan share with you that she saw this was a tissue of lies?

Def: I object.

Bill: Did she share that with you?

Def: I absolutely object. I object.

Cohe's truth remained behind the wall of objections. When Spa was asked about his involvement in the resident's neuro-consult note, he simply said, "it is signed by Dr. DeM," who, as it appeared, wasn't at the scene.

38

LIFELINE

MAY 5, 1997. A REMOTE PERSISTENT RING. Louder, now that I was awake. I'd arrived on a late-night flight for a morning meeting at the Montreal refinery with a fellow from France. "Are you sitting down?" Strange question. Gale knew I was sleeping. I couldn't be in any other position but supine, and in no other place but a downtown hotel, in the glow of a digital alarm clock showing 3:24 A.M. Her voice was calm, indicating the situation was tense, but eased. For sure, it had to do with . . .

Instantly, I sat up, fully alert, going over the recent events in my head.

Bobby had started his psych-ER rotation at the Clarke Institute of Psychiatry early in April—lectures in the mornings, patients in the afternoons that stretched to 7 P.M. Wheel Trans[22] was set up to take him to Clarke at College and Spadina, six blocks from Elm. But he had been wheeling over, mostly—in his own wheelchair—in order to get an extra hour of sleep in the morning. To avail himself of the transport, he had to be up at 7 A.M. But it took fifteen minutes of wheeling by himself, barring mishaps. Had it been a mishap, I wondered.

"No, not that," Gale repeated. Then what?

The Lifeline operator had called her 30 to 40 minutes before, and an ambulance had taken Bobby to the Mt. Sinai ER. He was disoriented when he arrived, but had improved as time progressed.

It was distressing. This type of thing seemed to be happening with increasing frequency, ever since the successful discoveries in Montreal.

PART 5: TORONTO, 1996

The dark of night began to fade away as daylight crept through the curtains. A disturbing thought appeared in my mind: had the seizures been causing falls, or the falls been causing seizures? Bobby's memory gaps made that determination impossible.

THE LATE AFTERNOON FLIGHT ON THE AIRBUS A320 WAS FULL. The agent gave me a bulkhead seat, even though I'd asked her not to when I changed my return flight for a stopover in Toronto. My computer couldn't be tucked under the seat in front: it had to ride somewhere else. I couldn't work—and it was work that sheltered me from worries of our shattered family, held together by grit and tenacity. I'd seen the face of the man next to me on the television before, one of the past premiers of Ontario. He said he was returning from a board meeting in Montreal—but I couldn't remember his name until he began to talk about his three bright children, ranging in age from 15 to 19. The youngest was a girl. I thought of Mon and Neilly. I'd missed Mon's med formal, and Neilly's parent-teacher interview. Bobby, the epicenter of the shatter, the demands of working for a living and the lawsuit drained away the days and kept me strapped, like the seatbelt on the bulkhead seat.

The door to Bobby's apartment was open when I arrived. Hospital security had brought Bobby back to his apartment. He was on the telephone, perhaps with Krista, asking for help. I took refuge in the next room. The table was out of place and the chairs scattered, one on its side on the floor, its back pointing toward the CD player by the wall. Bobby's eyeglasses were on the table. I waited until he got off the phone, and entered his bedroom.

A greasy REM hat loosely covered his long disheveled hair as he sat on his bed. A dark brown beard had grown to his chest and was starting to mat. I got near to take a closer look at a three-inch-long and two-inch-wide red scrape on his swollen forehead. There was also a wicked bruise over his right eyelid and a dangerous cut over the right eye.

"I told you not to come." He drew a difficult smile.

"How can I stay away? I took the day off tomorrow to attend Lee's discovery; I can skip it, if you want."

"Not a chance; I want you to see Dr. 'Decorticate' squirm." Bobby was firm.

"So do I," I said.

In fact, I'd checked my luggage through already, and had taken a cab from the airport on a four-hour stopover. Still, I would have changed my flight again, if Bobby had wanted me to.

"Krista will visit later."

"You want a drink for your meds?"

"Please."

The fridge was empty but for a lump of moldy cheese, a last glass of orange juice, and bottles, *not cans*, of pop that Bobby would have never bought. Someone I didn't know had been in. I brought him the glass of juice, sat down on his wheelchair—there was no other chair in the room—and watched him swallow the meds in one gulp. He lay down, hungry, exhausted.

As Bobby dozed off, I realized that I had no cash to buy him groceries, or time to cook food before the taxi would show up for my flight back to Calgary. I let Bobby sleep and headed out, in a hurry.

At the CIBC bank, at the corner of Dundas and University, a clerk had just closed the door and was about to step away. I knocked as I tried to catch my breath. "What do you want to do?" she asked.

"I need some cash for groceries."

She consulted with her colleague and opened the door just enough to let me in and I withdrew some cash. In a mad rush to the Hasty Market, I picked up some food. "Can you show me the ingredients of the sauce on the Bar-B-Q chicken?"

The clerk spoke little English and looked puzzled as she checked the Bar-B-Q machine and brought the empty gallon jug of sauce. "No nuts."

I skinned and washed all the sauce from the chicken despite the assurance, warmed up the ripped pieces, boiled some Brussels sprouts, carrots and potatoes, and served his dinner.

PART 5: TORONTO, 1996

"I didn't have anything last night, and had just a sandwich at lunch," he said as I helped him finish the food by his bedside. He wanted to be fed and needed help with his drink as well. His myoclonus shot up and he couldn't hold his glass steady. By the time I had cleaned up and put the leftovers away, the telephone rang; the cabbie was on time.

39

FELINE INSPIRATION

MAY 7, 1997. I HADN'T BEEN IN SADDAM'S PALACES, or in any other palace for that matter, but the stratosphere of the "Jewel of the West"—BJV's office floor—had the aura of a close second: palatial rooms, ornate furniture and luxurious bath and shower facilities. Lofty notary publics and patrons crossed over an extra-secure bank of elevators at this higher elevation. An overtly polite receptionist greeted patrons and clients as they stepped out above the clouds. I arrived early and was parked temporarily in a room.

Smartly dressed lawyers with dangling briefcases trailed by juniors with files under their arms started gathering in the opulent boardroom in a country club atmosphere. There were lawyers from MacKimmie Matthews for FHH, Parlee McLaws for JGH, and so on. I walked over to the boardroom, invisible to those around me, and pulled up a chair next to Bill. He'd strolled over from his office, a short distance away. I'd been there earlier to pick up the agenda of the discoveries and had learned that the Honorable Judge Pap had been appointed as the Case Management Judge. She'd meet with counsel from both sides on May 12. Coffee and refreshments were served with shiny silverware and fancy napkins, by the wall at the far end of the room, beyond the head table. I followed others, pouring coffee into a white china cup on a saucer. Dr. Lee arrived, tall, trim and dignified. His well-tanned face radiated smiles. He exchanged greetings and told stories of his visits to Nepal. And yet there seem to be an uneasy feeling that accompanied him and his theatrical appearance.

PART 5: TORONTO, 1996

"Your full name for the record, please?" Bill kicked off his examination of the 61-year-old veteran the moment a very diligent court reporter completed the swearing in, at 10:06 A.M. Bill and I were vastly outnumbered by the slew of defense lawyers.

The questioning went into high gear halfway through the afternoon, when Bill turned his attention to Lee's handwritten observation, examination and diagnosis on the morning following Bobby's arrival at FHH, sixteen days from Day Zero.

Bill: Well, let's just go to what you've written down here, page 25 of the clinical chart. Maybe we should just read the document together so that I understand your handwriting.
"Severe anaphylactoid reaction 16 days ago. Difficult intubation. Prolonged period of hypoxia, approximately one hour. Has remained comatose since. Was having myoclonic seizures, which were difficult to control but have now subsided. On 800 to 900 milligrams per day of Dilantin. Examination: Comatose. Trach. On ventilator. Frequent spontaneous flexion movement of both arms with intermittent extension of legs.? Decorticate."
What did you mean by that word?

Lee: The term "decorticate" or "decorticate posturing" is used to describe a situation in—either spontaneously or in response to stimulation—a comatose patient produces flexion movements of the arms and extension movements of the legs.

Bill: I take it the word suggests that there isn't a cortical involvement in terms of movement in those types of patients. Is that right?

Lee: The terminology arises from experimental work on cats, where if you remove the entire cerebral cortex and leave the rest of the brain intact, they exhibit this type of posturing.

MEDICAL MALADY

Bill: And so you questioned from your examination whether or not there was an involvement of the cortex in terms of the motor action that you observed in Bobby. Is that fair?

Lee: Yes.

A diagnosis, in his words, was based on experimental work on cats, from a veteran neurologist who'd earlier dismissed a neuropathologist's work on rats, saying, "…his work is based entirely on observations on rats, so that any interpretation of—or recommendation concerning—humans has to be extrapolated, because a human brain is very different from a rat brain."

He hadn't asked me for my input before putting his pen to the chart with that diagnosis—a diagnosis trailing a question mark that became definitive. If he had, I would certainly have said, prove it before putting it down on paper. But I know he would have probably been too quick at the draw to dismiss me, as nearly all of Bobby's doctors had. The three pillars of patient care—physician, patient and family—had all been missing, but not the cortex. All they had needed was the consent of two doctors—one as naïve as the R1 resident, even—to confirm the diagnosis. The other was left up to Sand, who was to take the witness stand next.

40

AMEND

THE ANTICIPATED DAY OF DARKNESS ARRIVED. Medium height, stocky, beard neatly trimmed, Dr. Sand, 54, director of the intensive care unit, professor and head of the division of critical care, University of Calgary, arrived at BJV's boardroom with his counsel, Quigley. He was duly sworn in by Valeara Gordon, court reporter, at 10 A.M., Thursday, May 15, 1997. The impressive position and imposing presence of the one who'd decided who would live and who would be denied didn't deter Bill from firing indignant queries. "Now, what about your certification? Are you certified in the area of critical care?"

> Sand: Actually, in Canada, there has never been a certification of just—so I can explain that for you. The Royal College of Physicians and Surgeons has a program called accreditation without certification," which means that they review the content of the program and assure that it is up to their standards, but there is no certifying exam, and all the trainings have their fellowships already.

I'd expected that doctors who make life and death decisions daily would be certified yearly. I'd thought that their power would be based on tested knowledge, skill, lifelong training and competence, and not on politics, position or prejudice. Seemingly not so. My attention turned back to the questioning.

Bill: And can you think of any clinical rationale why the Dilantin level wouldn't have been checked on the morning of the 18th after the change in dosage?

Sand: The primary rationale would be that the working diagnosis was status myoclonus, not generalized seizures.

Status myoclonus would be consistent with a decorticate cat. Admitting seizures would be admitting to a functioning cortex.

Bill: . . . did you assume that this patient, for example, had the capacity to sleep?

Sand: I think that, given his neurological status, it would be hard to define exactly what that state would be.

Admitting sleep would also have meant admitting to a functioning cortex. But Sand had something else in mind, something that had prompted him to dismiss the resident, the nurse's notes, and the Montreal neurologist:

Bill: Well, his resident, or the resident that accompanied him on rounds, records in her progress note that that was the rationale for continued dosage. And I can find it for you. Page 58 of the chart, bottom of the page, about the tenth line: "Continuing Dilantin 300 mg plus 60 mg IV phenobarb. Remains at risk for seizures." Do you see that note?

Sand: Mm-hmm.

Bill: So I'm just suggesting to you that the clinical rationale for continuing a dosage of Dilantin was that the patient was perceived to be at risk of seizure. Is that not fair?

Sand: No, that's not fair.

Bill: So, was this drug being administered, then, as a prophylactic against the possibility of epileptic seizure?

Sand: At that point, it was being administered as a remnant of a futile therapy for status myoclonus.

PART 5: TORONTO, 1996

Bill: Let's consider for a moment what Dr. Scho said. There was a component of this movement disorder, which he attributed to cortical epilepsy. What period of time would raise a concern for you, as an intensivist dealing with convulsant patients post hypoxic ischemic event, for that epileptic episode to continue?

Sand: First of all, there was no evidence to support Dr. Scho's clinical opinion. Secondly, the therapy, which he applied, did not change it. Thirdly, we had a strong clinical diagnosis of status myoclonus.

Sand, as it appeared, remained in status. Clinical diagnosis of a neurologist was dismissed as mere clinical opinion; whereas diagnosis of an intensivist—accredited without certification—ruled, sans definitive tests, that stopped lifesaving anticonvulsants. I wondered how they remained in business. Who would find out anyway? Lawyers seem to be in business for themselves; the court reporter recorded the charade:

Bill: Did you ever suggest to [Bobby's father] that if Bobby had a heart attack, no effort would be made to revive him?

Sand: It's our routine in our hospital that we have three—actually four—levels of care. They're called resuscitation status. It's expected that attending physicians discuss resuscitation status with all families or their proxies, and I did that as part of my routine.

Bill: So did you ever tell [Bobby's father], then, that the resuscitation level that Bobby was going to come under was one where if he had a heart attack you wouldn't revive him?

Sand: I raised this as a possibility. And there are three other levels: One is level 1, which is to do that plus all measures; 2 is all measures except CPR; level 3 is comfort measures only; and level 4 is brain death.

Stunned, I listened. I had no knowledge of this, these four levels of care. If I had, I would've known what level decorticates would've fallen into, and why Sand had given me the Wijdicks article. To them, Bobby was dead—brain dead.

The deposition ended at 3:21 P.M. with an exasperated parting shot from Bill. "I think we've been around the mulberry bush on that a bit already." We'd gone round and round on the same theme, of euphemisms, hiding behind undertakings, mixing times and facts, or resorting to amnesia. "I simply can't remember." Sand's lofty presence suddenly had no clothes. Shocks and shivers. More lay in wait.

PART 6:
SASKATOON, 1998

41

AURA

THE CALGARY DISCLOSURES WERE IN FULL SWING. Small fry—irrelevant in establishing liability—were being discovered for information on the big fish, and new names were being added to the claim. Work travels kept me away for some of the discoveries that I'd wanted to attend. Fraud charges leveled against Bobby by one of the government departments consumed my time, when time was in short supply. As if the fraud charge wasn't enough, Family and Social Services sent threatening letters. If $12,000 wasn't paid up in full immediately, they would send the files to a collection agency. We were being squeezed from every direction, it seemed. Perseverance prevailed, however. Bobby was in the middle of getting his career back, and carried on with his treatments.

THE SUCCESS OF THE DISCOVERIES RAINED A DELUGE of demands on us through defense lawyers, in unaccustomed jargon: Offers of Judgment, settlement without prejudice and the like, including one from Roon, Jen's lawyer. Her statement of defense had a new twist. She admitted to calling the Chinese restaurant from the apartment on Day Zero—a fact she'd denied previously. The story that Bobby was poisoned by Chinese food, as it turned out, was a red herring. However, the civil case against the hospitals was sealed. Calling it "a perfect legal case," Bill was prepared to cut Jen loose. The concern he posed was new: She would testify that Bobby was careless. The judge and the public would sympathize with the girl who had sat at

PART 6: SASKATOON, 1998

Bobby's bedside. The truth would remain hidden behind her bawling eyes, drawing sympathy and damaging credibility. Bill would rather go after the doctors, the deep pockets. But Bobby pushed hard. He wanted to know her story under oath. Bill wrote to Marc: "He is eager to examine [Jen]. I will [make] every effort to schedule this examination for discovery as soon as possible." He was annoyed, but agreed, warning that she might inflict damage. As far as we were concerned, she'd done the damage already.

THE LAWSUIT MOVED TO HYPERPLANE AT WARP SPEED. Talks of backroom dealings became more than a whisper. Bobby's affidavit on Production in April had shown him as "one of the Plaintiffs" in the action. That was about to change. Attached to the affidavit was repackaged information that I'd produced in February in a binder, and more since then. One hundred and sixteen documents that included Bobby's academic achievements (from childhood to becoming a doctor), articles that I'd written or clipped from newspapers, income tax returns that I'd filed on his behalf, budgets I'd prepared for him for residency training, and neuropsych test results that outlined his current intellectual shortcomings—a tilt, exploitable. The repackaged documents were numbered with dividers and put in three-inch ring binders bursting at the seams for service on the defendants. A massive undertaking that generated massive disbursements, a gold mine for the lawyers, munitions for the defense, now multiplied in a feeding frenzy.

The lawyers met with a case management judge. I had little knowledge of what a case management judge did for living, but I felt the ground shifting with the goings-on. Immediately after the meeting, Bill asked to see my diary. It seemed to be a ploy, because he had it in his possession already. I reminded him. "Handwritten notes," he said. I didn't argue, but the diary was handwritten, and it was a privileged document between lawyer and client, and therefore off limit for the defense.

Marc was also concerned about the ruse, but Bill comforted him. "In respect of the last issue you raised, namely Bobby's knowledge of the current state of affairs, I have brought him up to date with everything." Still concerned, the lawyer called. If Bobby had a falling out with Bill, he said, he would see the case through alone. Bill's voice came on the speakerphone soon after.

"Are we having a fight?"

"No, are we?"

"Then what's he talking about?"

"Send me a copy of his paper before you sign it."

A sure bet—the case that is. Both lawyers knew it, or they wouldn't have been jockeying for control.

"What do you think he's worth to us?"

"Around 10–15%."

"If the judge rules the trial to be held in Quebec, his worth goes up substantially."

The conversations could have been orchestrated as much for Marc as they were for me, I sensed, and the architect couldn't be Bobby. With all his disabilities, falls and fractures, he didn't have the energy or the legal smarts for the exchange—hockey scores, maybe, but not a lawyer's subterfuge. Bobby knew just enough to play by the script.

There were early signs that the lawsuit would settle long before the case would go to trial. It was just too scandalous for the defendants. As for Marc, he was as much a sucker as I was. Bill held all the cards. That made Marc queasy about the prospect of being left out. He'd sent a fax to Bobby: "As for my office's professional fees, they are a percentage of Bill's, to be established between him and me. We have been running presently on a gentlemen's agreement and a handshake .... Notwithstanding this agreement with Bill, you must understand that you and my office do have a direct professional link, such as, should any problem ever arise between you and Bill, my office will not be barred from invoicing its fees to you."

Bill appeared upbeat. He quipped, "It's going to be as nihilistic as I think it's going to be."

The warning bells I'd heard along the way kept on ringing. He had asked for more and received more of our research reference articles

PART 6: SASKATOON, 1998

through Marnie, his beleaguered secretary: "The Practice Parameters on the Assessment and Management of Patients in PVS" from the American Academy of Neurology, "The Standards of Care in the Practice of Neurology and Bioethics for Clinicians," the *CMA Code of Ethics*, and so on. The lawsuit, on a winning platter, was "nearly sewn up," she said. Now, little more information was to be gained from us; what remained was our hard-earned money. Susan, the other secretary, had given me the schedule for the rest of the discoveries. Dr. Seshia's blistering expert report arrived shortly thereafter. It left little doubt that the Calgary doctors had "incriminated themselves in the medical records by violating every Canadian law of medical and social ethics and caused horrendous emotional trauma."

A ten-page form from a Toronto rehab management consultant—engaged to prepare "a full assessment of the cost of future care" that must be filed with the court in 1998—arrived as I dropped in on Bobby on my way back from a business trip to Chicago. Much of the information on the form centered on the current cost of care, the bare minimum that could be afforded at the time. The consultant, with a halo of superiority for "court experience" over her head, would take a few months to complete the work at the princely sum of $95 an hour.

Bobby was being worked on from many fronts. Word got around; he became the key to a pot of gold, a node in the network of those who provided service to personal injury victims with settlements on the horizon. Two Toronto social workers befriended him, took him to an Independent Medical Examiner hired by the CMPA lawyers—at the Etobicoke General Hospital. One introduced Bobby to a thirty-something personal trainer, built like a bouncer. He did home visits, $65 an hour, for mat exercises. He was signed on, but Bobby was in debt and couldn't pay. It didn't matter, he was told; he could pay at his convenience. The personal trainer described himself as a businessman and a "financial advisor."

JUNE 24, 1997, SASKATOON. THE 32ND MEETING OF THE CANADIAN congress of Neurological Sciences. Bobby took a flight from Toronto, and I drove up from Calgary to meet him at the airport and take him to the Sheraton Cavalier hotel for four nights. His mission was to present a couple of posters in the mornings, and mine was to help him do so and gather information on the latest treatment for his iatrogenic epilepsy. Bobby was starting to recognize the warning signs of the seizures that had been striking him unannounced. His last three were preceded by trembling hands and an aura that he could see on occasion. Still, he could do nothing to stop the twister.

Sporting a purple COMPANION badge, I ran into Dr. Seshia by the elevator. I invited him to visit Bobby. He accepted and showed up following his task at hand. I was astounded when he announced that he had been fired from his position as pediatric neurologist at the Winnipeg Children's Hospital, as of July 1, 1997. A letter from his department had arrived a week before, shortly after he submitted his expert report to Bill.

42

DEAD SURE

NOVEMBER 17, 1997, 8:37 A.M. I WAITED IN THE OFFICE OPPOSITE the elegant BJV boardroom, not at all sure if I'd be allowed in. Roon, Jen's lawyer, objected to my presence—a presence that would be "too intimidating" for his client. Hogwash, I said. Bill hadn't been present in Montreal, and Bobby had been in a coma. Gale and I offered the only continuity. Gale wasn't interested in looking at Jen's face, nor in facing the lawyers she despised, and yet we needed the unbiased truth, wanted to witness the body language. Anticipating such a roadblock, I'd prepared a long list of questions for the occasion and handed it over to Bill. The objection to my presence sustained, the reason became clearer as the discovery unfolded:

> Bill: Did you go back into the apartment after you went in and cleaned it up? Was that the last time you went in there?
>
> Jen: No. I went back—I think I slept there one night, maybe more, and I know I at least had to go back once to get some stuff for me, though I don't know if I actually went in at that time.
>
> Bill: So you were back in the apartment after you'd cleaned it out in terms of the garbage and the Chinese food?
>
> Jen: Yeah.
>
> Bill: Was there any trash after you moved back in there for a night or two?
>
> Jen: I don't remember.

MEDICAL MALADY

Roon: You mean did she create any trash, or did the trash not get picked up?
Bill: I just wondered if you created any further trash after you cleared out the apartment.
Jen: Well, I mean, probably a used Kleenex or something. I don't remember there being—
Bill: Did you have any meals there, do you remember?
Jen: I don't think so. I think we mainly ate out.

Bobby and Jen had arrived from Ottawa in the late afternoon rush hour, close to suppertime, on Day Zero. Her assertion that she and Bobby "mainly ate out" explained why Gale and I couldn't find any sign of Chinese food in the apartment. The source of the poison that day hadn't been the Chinese food at all. Bobby's flashback came to mind: "While his [Mark's] back is turned, Freda takes some peanuts from her pocket and chews them up and swigs the last of her glass of wine."

There were more moments in the deposition that stretched the truth and twisted it past the breaking point:

Bill: His [Bobby's] eyes weren't red, glassy?
Jen: It was dark in the car.

Miraculously, however, the darkness vanished in her answer to another question:

Bill: Now, did you watch him administer the EpiPen that you brought to him from his backpack?
Jen: No. I know he took it because I remember on the drive to the hospital looking over at his leg, and his thigh was bleeding from the injection."

She couldn't see Bobby's eyes in the dark—around 11 P.M.—but she was able to spot bleeding on his thigh from an EpiPen injection, one that hardly produces a drop of blood, never mind enough to be visible through his thick jeans. The testimony seemed to corroborate what her father had revealed in our last family meeting: she wasn't in the car.

But why, then, was she lying? The likely reason could be found in the next exchange:

Bill: Did you take a large box of medical books from Bobby's apartment in Montreal?

Jen: Bob asked me to… I mean, I have them still, actually, and tried to give them back to Bob—no, sorry, I don't have them still. He did get them back.

It is conceivable that she was certain that Bobby wouldn't live to need the box of expensive medical books he'd taken to Montreal for his residency training. So she simply helped herself. She didn't know, it seemed, that her father had returned them when she'd flown the coop.

The episode ended finally, shamelessly. Relieved, the defendants' "key witness" walked over to her well-connected mother. Bill emerged with other lingering lawyers, none in any hurry to leave. I followed him to the elevator—past the pairs of watchful eyes—and went to La Flammery, on 3rd and 7th; the lunch was on my AMEX. Bill had finished a trial Friday and had little time to prepare, he said. The insurance company for the Chinese restaurant was eager to settle to avoid legal bills. He was equally eager to let the key defense witness walk and blame it all on the restaurant, regardless.

43

LADYSHIP

SATURDAY AFTERNOON. Mon crashed on the aisle seat of the Boeing 767, an Air Canada flight, courtesy of another companion ticket that Gale had gladly parted with. Two back-to-back calls made Mon's day a punishing thirty-six-hours long. She'd worked hard over the past month, but seemed happy. The surgical unit at Toronto's Mt. Sinai Hospital accepted her as a serious student, and she them as a good place to train. Bobby was deep in sleep when we'd left his apartment to head home. His support worker, Darryl, was a couple of hours late, and Bobby's meds would've been late too if I hadn't been there. This didn't bode well for an epileptic. With Mon asleep, I had time to record and reflect on the goings-on: her growing up to be a doctor, Neilly poised to be an engineer, and our resources—tangible and intangible—drained away on Bobby, who during the same month had spent the first week in Toronto, the second week in Calgary, the third week in the hospital from a disastrous fall, and the fourth week confined to a wheelchair due to a knee injury and general unsteadiness.

There was little time to celebrate Neilly's math award at the University of Calgary—for being one of the top three scorers in the Cayley math contest during that first week. I took a red-eye flight to Toronto instead, on my way to Chicago, and arrived in Bobby's apartment around 7:30 in the morning. Bobby was waiting. I wheeled him to the Canada Trust at Dundas and University, and converted $10,000 I'd taken out of our bank account, in Bobby's name, to give to Bill. He wanted it that way—perhaps to conceal the source, me; Gale wasn't

PART 6: SASKATOON, 1998

aware. I thought nothing of decimating our savings: it was for Bobby, and we'd get it all back, as Bill had said, to the penny, as the settlement was on the horizon. " . . . damage is so deep that the defendants may capitulate and make an offer of immediate settlement." With each successful discovery, however, Bill's demands for "dough" to cover his expenses grew louder, although the lawsuit was to have been undertaken on contingency.

The week following, I landed at the Alberta provincial courthouse at 6th Ave and 4th St., room 403, and found myself observing the proceedings of Her Ladyship—as the lawyers addressed her—perched on the judge's chair, back to the wall. I'd never been to such a courtroom. This must be the case management judge, I reckoned, but why weren't they addressing her as "Your honor"? The puzzle remained unresolved as I scanned the rest of the courtroom. The court reporter at the floor level straight ahead was recording diligently. The odd couple—slim Bill and plump Jamie—was on the first bench to my right, facing the judge. To the left was the BJV lawyer—not the one whom Bill had looked for to lead the defense team (he was on vacation), but one named Galag. Next to him was the CRHA lawyer. On the bench behind Bill were Marc and Bobby, whom I'd picked up from the airport a couple of nights before, in high spirits. The CP flight he'd been on didn't serve peanuts five rows in front and five behind. Perhaps my peanut lobby had produced results beyond Air Canada. To the right were three other lawyers and another behind them, representing four other law firms defending a variety of adversaries. I was in the middle of the third bench: the originator—the one who'd funded the lawsuit from his solitary paycheck, obtained medical witnesses, provided case histories and all the documents, and was now acting as a sketch artist and trying to follow the fast-paced proceedings for posterity and fairness, all in a quest for the truth. The defendants knew me; they were aware of my presence and persistence in this case, but they appeared bent on isolating Bobby from the rest of his family. It was a ploy that hospitals were crafty in applying, all under the cover of privacy.

The proceedings were in full swing when I'd pushed Bobby's

MEDICAL MALADY

wheelchair into the courtroom at 11:15 A.M. We had been held up at the citizen's appeal hearing on the fraud charge against Bobby. We'd waited for one of the three members forming the quorum of the quasijudicial body, who didn't show. It became apparent, however, that the fraud charge emanated from a lack of cooperation from the CRHA—one of the defendants in the lawsuit. The committee had the authority to pardon the claimed amount, about $12,000, to help a handicapped professional get back to work. After all, if he had stayed home in Calgary instead of going to Montreal, he would have collected $70,000 in social assistance instead.

My thoughts snapped back to the courtroom as I heard the lawyer strenuously arguing to include a violation of the Canadian Charter of Rights and Freedoms[23] (CCRF) in the amendment motions to the Statement of Claim, since Bobby's right to life, liberty and security had been jeopardized, due to the defendants' prejudice and the apparent falsification of the medical records. What would flow out of the Charter was punitive and exemplary damages if the CCRF was breached; hospitals were simply an arm of the government. The defense argued that if wrongdoing was established, compensation would follow and the establishment of prejudice would not be necessary; besides, it might delay the compensatory process.

Armed with the evidence of alleged "lies, cover-ups and screw-ups" in the charts, Bobby had sworn an affidavit over the telephone on August 27. All medical information Bill had asked me for—from Bobby's birth to 1994—was ready. Two other motions were tabled before the judge: to apply Quebec law in Alberta—to avoid riding two horses at the same time—and to include a bunch more doctors who had crawled out of the discoveries and into the Statement of Claim. The Quebec lawyer, who'd arrived the day before, sounded upbeat. The nurses' discoveries had gone well, and he'd translated relevant parts from French to English for us.

At the end of the day, Bill didn't get to include the CCRF against the hospitals on the grounds that the "Amendment must not create injustice, embarrassment" and that the "Charter issue creates unnecessary

PART 6: SASKATOON, 1998

complications," but he won on another count: that the "case would be presented as a story against all defendants, not just the Montreal defendants or the Calgary defendants." Bill's concluding comment to the judge echoed in my ear: "The case is going extremely well in terms of collaborative effort." Did I hear "collaborative effort?" Soothing words for the judge, maybe, but a burning sensation descended on me. Any collaboration appeared to be a recipe for collusion.

Bobby returned to Toronto. Ethan, grown son of Gale's prenatal-class friend, and his new wife Margit had picked up Bobby from the airport. Four days later, Life Alert called. Around 1:45 P.M., Bobby had suffered a serious fall. He'd been found unconscious on the floor, bleeding. How long he had been there was a mystery. The blue curtain I'd installed—for Mon's privacy in the living room, where she slept in a sleeping bag—fluttered in the autumn breeze from open windows and had perhaps set off cortical reflex myoclonus. He'd spun around, fallen and passed out. He could describe exactly how it'd happened. That meant no seizure—not this time, or his memory would have been wiped out. Part of his hair and the skin from his left eyebrow remained on the curtain around the one-inch rip, courtesy of the sharp corner of the heating and air conditioning duct. When he'd regained consciousness, he'd depressed the Life Alert button for the paramedics to take him to the hospital for five stitches over one blackened left eye and a torn knee ligament. He remained in the hospital, needed help to bathe, and was ordered not to walk in the apartment.

EACH STEP SEEMED UPHILL, THE DAYS EXHAUSTING. I dragged myself to the BJV boardroom table on my return to Calgary and pulled up the chair next to Bill. I was invited back, alone, for the discovery of Dr. Panis. A puny player—an appendage of little significance in the larger scheme of things—he opted out of CMPA insurance and hired his own lawyer, or had one hired on his behalf. New faces, with half-eyes on their noses and wearing well-tanned skin from rich vacationland, spitting smart repartees from thin lips. Lean, mean looks, dollars in one eye and a question mark in the other, they raised their heads as I came through the door. They returned my glance around the table through the corner of their eyes, as if it was their bonanza—what in the world was I doing there. Middle-aged lead lawyers sat down, settled, and then scurried to be on the same page as their colleagues. They meant business. Juniors were in and out. Bill seemed to have gained new respectability—and a larger audience—with the arrival of the lead CMPA lawyer, the one he'd wanted, albeit delayed. He took the empty seat at the head of the table. Louise, the lead CRHA lawyer, and Norah, the lead JGH lawyer, were at their seats already. The appendage lawyers—Donald and Richard—appeared subservient to the lead CMPA lawyer. One of them, Donald, had written to Bill as far back as August 1997: "Although our client Dr. Panis is not presently a party to the Alberta litigation, our expectation is that we will be attending the examination in the capacity of observer."

The court reporter swore in Dr. Panis, and Bill went over the same mundane questions he'd repeated thousands of times before, or so it seemed. The game of objections and denials played out again ad nauseam. Sixteen pages of scribbles later, Panis's discovery ended for the day. The work would continue with Dr. Bern and the nurses at MacKimmie Matthews, in the Gulf Canada Building.

With a settlement near—an offer of $100,000 from JGH was being bandied about, perhaps an admission of sorts—the discoveries to follow seemed mere formalities. Louise and Bill apparently went to the case management judge. The details remained obscure, but I felt the effect: the duo succeeded in keeping me out. Bill said to me later, "Pisses me off; can't believe it." Yet, he wouldn't appeal, showing an incongruity between his words and his actions. I attended Bern's discovery, but was told I wouldn't be allowed in for the nurses'. Efforts on both sides were being made, I sensed, with the coming of the new CMPA lead lawyer, to exclude me from the discoveries. Leaving the seventh floor of the Gulf Canada Building, I stopped by Bill's office. Jamie had words of comfort: Most people can't start a lawsuit; they don't find the truth because they don't have the ability. "They get on with their lives, go to church and pray. They don't know what hit them."

PART 6: SASKATOON, 1998

We were not in that category: we knew what hit us. But what would hit us next, from those I'd hired to fight our lawsuit, remained a nagging concern.

44

SCROOGE

DECEMBER 21, 1997. ON THE SUNDAY MORNING BEFORE Christmas, our Oakfern kitchen was warm with activities. The children were home. Buttermilk pancakes bubbled on the nonstick skillet; breakfast was nearly ready. Neilly tiptoed to the round kitchen table where we'd sit in a circle on wooden stools, took a whiff of the flapjacks on his plate, and screamed in horror. "What did you put in it?"

I hesitated to give away the secret, but Neilly's nose couldn't be fooled: he hated banana in his pancakes. Bobby drooled over them; he'd started to eat one already, as if he hadn't eaten in days. Mon was in the middle. "It's okaaay, Neilly, try it," she said as she served him a glass of orange juice. Gale, busy pouring coffee, was enjoying the togetherness immensely. It meant much more now, since Bobby's injuries had transformed our lives. Despite the closeness, I could sense forces trying to tear the family apart.

The change had come surreptitiously. With each visit back to Calgary, as it appeared, Bobby was compelled to keep an appointment with the psychologist at the Foothills special services building. After each visit, like the battering of wind on a shoreline, a noticeable aloofness eroded his mind, orienting him away from the family. The visit this time had an added twist. Bill wanted to meet with him alone, on December 19, 1997, at 9 A.M. Carroll, his secretary called my office an hour later, asking me to join them.

A ransom chorus bellowed the moment I walked in: "Did you bring the dough?" Bill wanted a $400,000 war chest, and he needed 50,000

PART 6: SASKATOON, 1998

now. So close to a settlement, the urgency astounded me. I've used up my cash savings, I said. He asked for details of my finances: income, investments, RRSPs, rental properties. No free cash. Negative, I said.

"House?" he asked.

"Wife won't allow it."

Bobby joined in: You own half.

It didn't take long to realize that Bill had already covered these items with Bobby and had won him over. I agreed to pay $10,000 per quarter from my personal line of credit. I wondered whether it was to dollar us out, despite the contingency arrangement. But why?

THREE DAYS LATER, while pushing Bobby's wheelchair from the Home Oil Tower to the Banker's Hall for his discovery—Bobby had been declared the sole plaintiff, without any reference to the family—Bill broke the news. The lead CMPA lawyer had called him, he said. I wouldn't be allowed in for discovery; Bobby would have to manage on his own devices—meds and personal care included. Bill didn't want to go to the case management judge to plead our case. Shocked, I began to realize that scrupulous legal advice would have included all of our names in the lawsuit, either at the outset or in one of the amendments that followed. I sensed a horrible hoax, but it was too late to do anything about it now.

The discovery notes arrived days later. They read like an indictment against the entire family—medical, educational, and occupational histories were explored, with few objections thrown in the way. Irrelevant, incorrect information from an injured mind, fresh out of a debilitating coma, became part of the court documents. This wouldn't have been possible if we had been named. It was a perfect opportunity for the defense lawyers to grope for somebody—dead or alive—on whom to pin the blame: What about your grandfathers; do you know if they had any significant disease problems?

The lawyers took turns grilling Bobby, humiliating him with inappropriate questions: Sexual function? They pushed him for responses that were already in their medical examiner's report, without redress:

MEDICAL MALADY

"You don't know whether there is any sexual function at this time?"

The queries made me cringe and wonder why we had been told that Bobby's discovery wouldn't amount to much. The lawyers seemed to befriend him at one point, patronize him the next. Questions began or ended with "Sir," but then they talked down to him, changed tacks, or introduced detractions. In time, they discovered the poison—peanuts—and we the poisonings, not only on Day Zero, but at other times as well.

> Mart: What had happened, as best you can recall, leading to the 1993 hospitalization?
> Bob: What happened was Jen and I were eating dinner—or attempting to eat dinner at Buchanan's [restaurant in Calgary]. Apparently, Jen had some soup and I had another appetizer. Jen said, "Why don't you try my soup? And I tried a bit of her soup and I got a reaction to it right away.
> Mart: Is there a problem with, if you smell the odor of peanuts?
> Bob: Yes.
> Mart: If you inhale that smell, does that cause any reaction at all?
> Bob: That might.
> Mart: Would that be something that certainly by June of 1994 you were able to identify just on a straight odor basis; you had a strong sense that there might be nuts in something?
> Bob: No. No. You would have to have peanut butter, all right, in my face for me to pick up the odor; or you would have to have me playing and everyone around me eating nuts for me to pick up the odor. Okay? But say, for example, if it's in a sauce or disguised in sauce, it's disguised in a soup, I wouldn't pick up the odor.

An opportune moment arrived for the defense to push forth a distraction.

> Mart: "Well, I thought this whole lawsuit was about peanut allergies."

PART 6: SASKATOON, 1998

To let the notion pass without challenge would let them get away with the medical blunder that had bludgeoned Bobby into a coma. Bill retorted: "I thought this lawsuit was about medical malpractice."

The line of questioning was switched to relationships:

Mart: Up to June 30, 1994, can you describe the nature of your relationship with your father?

Bill: Relevance?

Mart: Well, his father seems to have been, naturally enough, heavily involved in all aspects of the treatment from June 30 on for a considerable period of time. I'd just like to know what the relationship was between the father and the son.

Bill: I think it's irrelevant. The only issue arises as to who was Bobby's proxy, and you have the admission from all the medical doctors, that *his father* is Bobby's proxy.

The discharge note from FHH also illustrated attempts to vilify me—labeling me as "difficult to deal with" and "unable to accept Bobby's prognosis." Clearly they'd identified me as one who'd likely push for the patient's rights and well-being, one who would uncover wrongdoings had there been any—and there had been many more than one, they knew. They also knew that damaging notes against me, useful in a lawsuit, would be written by a resident who'd depart following his or her rotation, leaving the staff doctors free and clear. I began to see the rationale for marginalizing Gale and me that began at JGH with Dr. Spa, was carried on at FHH, and was continuing to this day.

Mart: Have you asked your father about discussions he has had with Jen—arising out of the events on June the 30th?

Bob: Yes.

Mart: What did he tell you?

Bob: He said that there were some activities that he wasn't sure of that were—that he was uncertain of.

Mart: What activities were those?
Bob: For the first three or four days, he, I believe, trusted Jen, and then after that she started acting like a medical resident, or what have you, and I believe the rest of that is—I know there's, in the United States, spousal privilege. I don't know about the law in Canada, but my discussions with my father are private.
Mart: What in particular had been objectionable?
Bob: Calling in her mother, her father, her aunt; giving presents to Dr. Spa, like scotch, after I left; and influence peddling between—or splitting between the doctors, my family, and her family was objectionable, and was not right.

The defense frustrations showed. They would keep changing tactics and strategy until the bond between the proxy and the victim would be broken, the victim corralled.

Mart: Sir, each time you editorialize in one of your responses, you add to the length of this discovery. Sir, what is your—
Bob: Was that a question?
Mart: I made an observation. What is your understanding as to how your injuries occurred?
Bill: What injuries?
Mart: The injuries that we've been discussing for the last day.
Bill: What injuries?
Mart: The injuries arising out of the incident in June and July of 1994.
Bob: That's a complicated question. I believe I had poorly treated anaphylaxis—anaphylactic shock—as well as poorly treated status epilepticus, which has caused the brain damage that I have.

PART 6: SASKATOON, 1998

Time period specified, Bobby aptly encapsulated the injuries that were inflicted upon him. A hint of the injuries that awaited us came on Christmas Day. Our lead medical witness—who'd lost his position with the Winnipeg hospital—lost his appeal to get his job back as well.

45

PRIVATE EYE

JANUARY 23, 1998, 11:34 A.M. BILL BROKE AWAY from the middle of a meeting he was attending, to call me at work. Voice firm, he warned, "No contact with the Crown, cease and desist writing to the police." If the discoveries confirmed unlawful acts, we'd go to the police and to the Crown with the documents, as we'd discussed at the outset. Jamie had couriered copies of some of the discovery notes. Previously, we'd been called to pick them up. The meeting Bill broke away from seemed to have changed all that, triggering something sinister.

The turn of events was heightened by Bobby's call a few days later. Confused and non-communicative, he wanted Mon's telephone number. He didn't seem to remember where she was, although I'd told him that we'd helped her move from Edmonton on the first of the month. She was adjusting to her new life in Rimbey—a tiny town of 2,000 in Alberta—where she had to complete a month of mandatory family medicine clinic before graduating. Soon to be a doctor, she would practice under the protection of the hospitals and the government, supported by the doctor's insurance company, the CMPA. She'd already been adversely affected by the turn of events and sacrificed plenty, and now the new development became a matter of concern, as it had the potential to pose a threat and set her off course.

Bobby called again days later, Bill soon after. The message was the same: Bill didn't represent me, *the proxy*. Surprised, I interjected, "I beg your pardon. Why would I need representation?" We had one lawsuit—the family's. I'd hired Bill to look after it, and the family had

PART 6: SASKATOON, 1998

provided funds, searched witnesses, dug out all the information, and given support. That made the case winnable enough for Bill to take it up on contingency. Bobby was named the only plaintiff to avoid complexity, and conserve resources. But the story took a crooked turn.

A wiry, middle-aged woman in slacks and a spring jacket leaned against the wall by the elevator bank on the seventeenth floor of my office building, clutching a manila envelope. She approached me as I got off one of the elevators, ready to thrust the envelope into my hand. I wasn't about to accept it without an explanation. I swiped my ID card and held the door open. She hesitated, but came into the hallway and followed me into my office. Gale's description of a woman who had visited Oakfern a couple of days earlier, and asked her to surrender my diary, didn't match the description of the one who sat cross-legged at the edge of the only chair across from my desk. She was polite, almost apologetic, as she placed the envelope on my desk and retracted her hands to clasp between her knees, ready to answer questions.

Marnie, as she introduced herself, had been tracking me for a couple of days, from the James Short underground parkade across 5th Ave to my office in PC Centre. I matched the profile she had been given. She'd do whatever they wanted done—she needed the money.

I asked, "Who are they?"

Her answer astounded me. She was employed by a private investigator, Backtrack, hired on by Donald, one of the appendage lawyers hired by Dr. Panis. We didn't need him—he'd probably be allowed to walk without liability—and yet his lawyer had invited himself into the defense team.

An affidavit was in the envelope that Marnie left behind. It seemed to have been drawn up at the advice of Louise, the lead lawyer for FHH, and it bore the signature of John, a senior officer of the CRHA. It legitimized not the fact that I'd kept a contemporaneous diary of events, but that John had personal knowledge of it.

Attached to the affidavit were two letters: one by the lead CMPA lawyer, Mart, asking Bill to provide my notes. The other was Bill's response that he was unable to comply, for, he reasoned, I was not his client. That flew in the face of his acquiring the electronic copy of my diary in Montreal—by asserting that there shouldn't be any secret between client and solicitor—and my endless dealings with him; he'd given me receipts for payments I made to him in my name. However, it did explain the reason he'd asked that the $10,000 I paid to him last, to be made out as if Bobby was paying him. A medical malpractice lawyer in close collaboration with the defense, close to a settlement, could pick and choose his client, or my diary would be a privileged document, out of bounds for the defense.

Bill's denial caught me by surprise, made me a target. It was an open invitation for the defense team to attack me, the one who had uncovered the wrongdoings and had brought a lawsuit against the powerful defendants. Suddenly, the prophetic remark of the Ultramont anesthesiologist, and the warning of the San Francisco neurologist—our quest for truth behind the curtain of internal hanky-panky in Canada would be no less traumatic than the injuries that had necessitated it—began to ring true.

MARCH WITNESSED MYRIAD CHANGES in Bill's office. Two new secretaries arrived, Joan and Susan, fresh from BJV's offices. The ones who'd known me were gone. Joan, quick-witted, tall and slender, took charge of the case full time. She informed me that Bill had been looking for me prior to the nurses' discoveries at MacKimmie Matthews in the Gulf Canada building. I was out of my office. In fact, my current projects, scattered nationally, were keeping me busy.

Joan called on me on March 18 and instructed me to attend a meeting with the case management judge the next day. It was scheduled to start at 8 A.M., but I was to be there at 11. Mind preoccupied—impending merger talks between Ultramar and PCA were creating upheaval on the work front; a layoff, or a transfer back to the office in Toronto were real possibilities—I took the C-train to the Alberta provincial courthouse at 6th and 4th. The lawyers, huddled in front rows, had already been meeting with the judge for three hours. I could see Mart (BJV, representing CMPA—the doctors), Ken (Parlee McLaws,

PART 6: SASKATOON, 1998

representing JGH), Roon (Roon Prentice, representing Jen), Louise (MacKimmie Matthews representing FHH and Scott, a resident) and Don (Burnet Duckworth & Palmer, representing Panis). Bill was among them now, part of them. I couldn't tell.

I stood alone, stood up. What was happening seemed fictional, fraudulent even, but very real. Suddenly, the judge lifted her head, looked in my direction, and said something in haste. What did she say? My mind was too boggled to interpret it. Where was my affidavit? Was I supposed to have one? She didn't seem to have any patience. She ordered me to produce one by March 26, and moved to the next topic, whatever it was. I suppose I needed to hire another one of those folks who take suckers for a ride.

It was a brief appearance in the courtroom; I was dismissed before I could say more. My departure went as unnoticed as my arrival, or so I thought. But someone had noticed. As I arrived back at my office, I looked over my shoulder. There was Marnie, the private detective. She seemed to have followed me from the courthouse.

46

BLUFF

MARCH 23, 1998. THE BRENTWOOD C-TRAIN TURNED northward as it took the trajectory of the tracks over the Bow River, squealing. I was shunted off in that direction to see another lawyer, Allen. Bill seemed to have already talked to him.

Allen looked much younger than he'd sounded over the telephone: pleasant, no four-letter words, not hardened, or so it seemed. He advised me to hand over the diary to the judge—the diary that I had given Bill in 1996 when I'd first met him, and that Bill had retrieved from his files and tossed back to me in his office before getting hold of Allen.

"Then why do I need to hire you?"

"To write the affidavit."

Of course. I wrote him a check. He wouldn't spend the entire amount of $1000, he said. *Haven't I heard that before?* I hadn't told Gale I was meeting him after work. She'd find out anyway; she reconciled our decimated bank account. Why did I need a second lawyer, she'd ask, when I'd just paid the first one yet another ten grand? She'd reminded me, over and over again, that to trust a Calgary lawyer was to trust fangs and a forked tongue that spat out confusion, not clarity. She had a point: Bill's statement of account continued to show me as his client in Montreal and Calgary, and I received any and all documents related to Bobby's case.

A HEAVY SPRING SNOWFALL BLANKETED TORONTO over the weekend. With no caregiver, no food, and no one to help, Bobby

PART 6: SASKATOON, 1998

managed a pizza delivery for supper Sunday night. That was all. I called Loblaws at Dupont and Christie on Monday morning and faxed a shopping list from Calgary—to have nut-free groceries delivered to his apartment—as I left home for a meeting in Edmonton.

In the middle of the meeting, the refinery secretary signaled from the door for me to pick up the telephone in the next room. An unmistakable accent caused me to shake in anticipation. If the merger with Ultramar were to go through, I would be transferred to Toronto, along with a hundred others. Most weren't keen to move. The merger hadn't happened, spilled the accent. So, why the call? "I have good news and bad. The good first: you still have a job; the bad: it's not in Calgary."

"Toronto?"

"Yes."

"E-e-e-yes!" I surprised him, and myself as well, nearly throwing the telephone up in the air. Do I mind? Hell no, not at all. Although it'd mean a weekly commute between the two cities, until Neilly graduated and enrolled in Waterloo, our move would help Bobby stave off crises like the one this morning. Mon would soon relocate to start her residency at Ottawa General—within driving distance of Toronto.

WEDNESDAY, JUNE 17. Bill wrote to ask me to pick up the final set of transcripts from the discoveries completed in Montreal for review. Bobby had reportedly signed a waiver—one of many papers he told me he'd signed—for Bill to negotiate with the Chinese restaurant. Overtures had apparently been made for settlement. The Quebec City lawyer's letter in May seemed to have scared them into submission, as chatters could be vaguely overheard in the lawyer's offices:

"The two girls from Bennett Jones had not seen anything like this before..."

"This case consumed my life; we found the largest mallet we could find..."

"CMPA had a powwow after the case management meeting . . . where finger pointing took place that would lead to a fight between defense counsels, apportion the blame . . ."

"Ken, John, Louise were all there...They'd find experts to point fingers elsewhere . . ."

"We managed to hook someone . . ."

The telephone rang off the hook all day; the CMPA secretary called Joan: "My, you were busy!"

The Quebec City lawyer's letter to the Chinese restaurant's insurance company had cast the hook: ". . . The whole story starts at the restaurant. Depending on the judge's view of the case, the liability issue can end at the restaurant or keep on going at the hospital and involve the doctors and the personnel. One thing is for sure: we can count on defendant hospitals and doctors to adduce evidence that Bobby's actual and permanent catastrophic condition has nothing to do with whatever co-defendants did or did not do and everything to do with the anaphylactic reaction caused by the ingestion of peanuts. This defense clearly puts the focus on the alleged restaurant's negligence . . ."

Though the evidence showed otherwise, it didn't stop the mallet from being wielded. ". . . I am also told that the Alberta rules provide that an official request for payment of the limits can be brought up and, if it is not accepted, the insurance carrier can be forced to pay the whole amount of damages if, eventually, liability is found against the insurance carrier."

Then it cajoled: ". . . What do we do about this whole situation? We think that from an insurance company's point of view, the disbursement figures and the risk of being caught for a substantial amount over the actual limit of the policy are so high, a deal—any deal—is a good one. Mind you, I talked separately to Mr. Mc and Mr. M and Mr. B, and each of us came to the same conclusion that it would be sound business for an insurance carrier to put its limit on the table. This also has the advantage of rendering useless any warranty suit the co-defendants might want to bring against the restaurant . . ."

It appeared to be a gargantuan bluff. Had the poisoning taken place at the restaurant, anaphylaxis would've been instantaneous—nothing short of injecting an EpiPen could have forestalled its wrath.

PART 6: SASKATOON, 1998

Nor was there a shred of evidence of Chinese food in the apartment, though the poison had certainly been there. And that pointed to the source: Jen. The Chinese restaurant didn't know that; neither did they have Jen's deposition, apparently.

Bill's Montreal trip—following a detour through Winnipeg for consultation with the now unemployed star medical witness—concluded the discoveries of the remaining doctors, residents and ICU nurses, and tied up the loose ends. All of them were reported to have "contradicted each other" under oath. The resident, least prepped of all, was reported to have told nearly the whole truth—foreign to the prepped witnesses. But none testified to the demon—the one who actually inserted the NG tube without checking its placement—who sucked Bobby's life right out of his body and left him to die.

47

DOUGH BOY

OCTOBER 21, 1998, 1:20 P.M. BUFFY CALLED ME AT THE REFINERY, his voice panic-stricken: "Bobby is not responding!" A seasoned caregiver from the Spectrum Health Care agency, Buffy had become a trusted friend who often went beyond the call of duty. His wife was a nurse at Mt. Sinai.

"Is he dead? Is he breathing?" I blurted out in terror.

"No, he is breathing, but he seems to be in a coma . . . how long will it take you to get here?"

I asked him to remain with Bobby, alerted the nurses' station on the 17th floor of the situation, and rushed out of the trailer—our temporary office in Oakville, by the odorous API[24] separator. I walked as fast as I could to the main gate to be waved off, and then ran to the packed parking lot in search of my car. "Not again," I heard myself repeating to my pounding heart. "Not again."

The ward nurse had responded calmly. "Don't panic; he is just sleeping." I wouldn't have, if it wasn't Buffy who'd called, and if the specter of past emergencies had faded from my memory. The sequence of events leading to this episode kept on playing in my mind on the drive that took nearly an hour through the thick Queen Elizabeth Way traffic.

The appointment of the mediator had been announced in September 1998, following a flurry of reports and rebuttals. BJV had ordered yet another neuropsych test, as if the battery of testing that preceded it wasn't draconian enough. There had been three separate

PART 6: SASKATOON, 1998

ones already: first by FHH, next by BJV, and the one after was ordered by Bill. Each had been a two-day torture for Bobby.

A week prior to this day, Bobby had wheeled six blocks to the Clarke and then returned to Mt. Sinai so that Helen—a new friend, a psych nurse—could give him a ride to the multidisciplinary assessment center on Dufferin for the tests ordered by BJV. A neuropsych, two psychs, and an occupational therapist took turns for two days, he said. The neuropsych "pushed him to the brink," from 9:30 A.M. to 6:30 P.M., with virtually no break on the first day. He suffered a seizure and a fall, which left a bad bruise on his elbow that had been examined in the Mt. Sinai ER that very night. He was ordered back the next day regardless, for another battery of tests. This time it was with the psychs and the OT. Post-medical report, the CMPA scheduled him for another discovery session in December. It seemed to confirm the notion that they wanted to break him before the judicial dispute resolution (JDR), which Joan confirmed was to be held February 1–5, 1999.

I hurried to the hospital room at 2:28 P.M. A swarm of white coats was leaning over Bobby—still unconscious, lying on his back, face up, with froth rolling down the side of his mouth and over his thick black beard. The pulse oximeter read 76%, significantly lower than the normal 90%. I gasped—as if I'd changed places with him—and yelled at the resident to get the ICU resident, to get the saturation up. With gadgets in hand, the ICU resident arrived, nervously hesitating to intubate. She cried out in panic: "I wish Dr. Mitchell was here." That very moment, the doc wandered in, hands in his white coat pocket. Calmly, he took hold of the ET tube by the head of the bed. The resident opened Bobby's mouth with the scope and I opened mine. Bobby's head thrust backward, throat up, Dr. Mitchell said, "I can't see yet." The resident exerted some more thrust, the ET tube was inserted, and the respiratory therapist (RT) began squeezing the oxygen bag. Within a minute, his saturation magically moved up to 81%. Dr. Mitchell handed over the patient and walked off at 2:38 P.M., the same way he walked in, with a relaxed confident stroll. I began breathing again.

Bobby was moved to the ICU. His blood sample, the nurse said, was like "cheese." The laboratory results arrived, with a triglyceride level reading 88 mmol/l—forty-four times higher than normal—pointing to a damaged pancreas.

A balding, average-sized man in his forties approached and politely introduced himself as I was talking to Gordon, the neurologist. He was the ICU chief, minus the haughty disposition we'd been accustomed to. He seemed eager to piece together what had made Bobby comatose again. Helen walked into the conversation, and filled in the details. Stomach pain had started in the evening and had escalated following the ER admission. Shortly after the nurse administered 75 mg Demerol and 50 mg gravol—perhaps an overdose of Demerol—he vomited, and a seizure of short duration ensued at 2 a.m. An hour later, at Helen's repeated request, he was moved to a resuscitation room and hooked up to oxygen. She decided to remain with him through the night, on pins and needles, until he was transferred to Room 1715 in the South Wing at daybreak.

Satisfied that Bobby would live, saved by the diligence of Helen and Buffy, I decided to visit his apartment in search of food. I hadn't been in the apartment since my office had been relocated from Calgary in September, and I'd moved to Arista Towers, a company-sponsored condo close to my office. Like a mole, I took the underground utility tunnel that joined the hospital to the apartment building and went up the elevator to Bobby's 10th floor residence. Hamburgers, nothing but hamburgers. The fridge was stuffed with them—in lunch boxes and in dinner packs. It would have taken me weeks to eat my way through the cooked fatty patties. He had been eating this, I reckoned, for days and nights. "Why?" I asked aloud. "Why are the cupboards infested with little roaches that weren't there before?"

The answer came as Bobby got better over the next eighteen days of hospitalization, days that lowered his triglycerides to 5.36 mmol/l with ever more drugs added to his daily dosettes: for high lipids, wild fluctuations in blood sugar, absence seizure (seizures without external symptoms) and PVC (premature ventricular contractions). Despite

PART 6: SASKATOON, 1998

becoming an insulin-dependent diabetic, along with other ailments that required considerable attendant attention, people found him a delight to be with and Helen's relationship with him deepened. She remained with him nearly every day until I got there at night.

The impending JDR had brought out the smell of money for others. It was outlined in the Long-term Functional Needs and Costs Analysis report: "The costs outlined in this report reflect extraordinary costs, specifically those that would not be incurred had he (Bobby) not sustained these impairments." Every decade he lived would require a baseline cost of $1.35 million to $1.52 million. Strange visitors appeared out of the medical–legal woodwork, setting off a flurry of competing activities for his care and well-being. One of the two Toronto social workers who had befriended him when the cost of future care was first estimated apparently brought in a proposal for Bobby to be a male figure in the lives of a couple of eighteen-year olds attending a remedial school. One of the boys' father had left, his mother committed suicide and he went to live with the other boy's mother, whose husband had left. The three of them offered to cook for Bobby in return for his presence in the boys' lives. Bobby had apparently accepted their proposal without background checks or agency referrals. By mid-September, the boy's mother had assumed the position of Bobby's surrogate mother, squeezed out the caregivers and begun cooking for him.

At about the same time, Jen's "best friend," who'd visited Bobby in Montreal and held the wake in Calgary in 1994, showed up at his doorstep seeking shelter, reacquainting through a shared hockey pool. The Toronto social worker, Joan the secretary, and the friend twittered in a patronizing tune; Bobby needed female company. But then, he had Helen. To that, the nefarious friend chimed, "Bobby, you deserve better," and moved in, with her large stuffed suitcase in tow. She began using his computer and email, as if she were on a mission to encircle the "dough boy." Since his hospitalization, however, the army of surrogates that had marginalized the caregivers had retreated.

48

SQUEEZE

IT WAS DECEMBER 1998 WHEN BOBBY, ON THE MEND yet again, was scheduled to start work at the Hospital for Sick Children, in Toronto, following the New Year's holiday. Bill had been preparing for mediation as the reports—the plaintiff's expert statements, the defense's expert statements, and the plaintiff's rebuttal of the defense expert statements—rolled in. Mon was settled in Ottawa in residency training. Gale was devoted to her work and to Neilly, and counting the weeks until she could leave Calgary permanently, to be closer to Bobby. I shuttled between the cities over the weekends, and between Bobby's apartment and mine, just twenty minutes away in Mississauga, on weeknights.

It seemed order had taken hold in our lives amid the chaos. Then, one afternoon, Bobby informed me that Marc had quit, and that Bill was looking for a co-counsel to replace him. I recalled that Bill had mentioned to me at the outset that Brian, our first lawyer in Calgary, had worked as his co-counsel on another case prior to ours, involving a settlement of a million and a half. Brian apparently declined to be his co-counsel this time around. Perhaps he'd sensed from his experience that something wily was in the works. Why else would a supporting actor who'd done everything to make the case a success quit before the final act? The Quebec City lawyer wouldn't return my call.

I decided to call his anesthesiologist father, a convivial doctor with whom I had had congenial conversations in the past. But not this time. Marcel's tone was sour. "Marc didn't drop out of the case,

PART 6: SASKATOON, 1998

you must know." No, I didn't. He calmed down when he heard our story—milked endlessly, then sidelined with another lawyer, costing more, as Bill's demands continued to escalate. Apparently, Marc had been given notice to move to Calgary and spend six months there for "the trial," an imposition that was impossible for him and his young family to fulfill. Bill let him go. Marcel thought I'd had a hand in Marc's firing. Puzzled, I asked, "What trial?" The mediator, a retired judge from Victoria, had already been appointed. The talk of a trial sounded like the ploy of a pirate closing in on a pot of gold. Two down and one to go.

I DIALED THIRTY UNITS OF INSULIN NPH INTO THE SYRINGE. The St. Elizabeth nurse who visited Bobby in his apartment four times a day, for his doses of insulin, hadn't shown up. Bobby took the syringe out of my hand, waited until the shaking stopped, jabbed the needle into his stomach, and started to push with his thumb. Before he could finish, the next onslaught of myoclonus jerked his hand and dragged the needle across his belly, opening a long razor-sharp gash that instantly turned bloody. I thought the needle had broken and lodged in his flesh, but it hadn't. It had simply bent a little, and the plunger remained stuck at 23. His face showed signs of defeat. He had no idea how much insulin had gone into his body.

"Why in God's name did you want to do it yourself?" My patience had worn thin. I had injected him many times before, when the nurse or his attendant hadn't shown, but times were changing.

"They want me to take two months off . . . learn to live with my diabetes, on my own." The two months coincided with the JDR.

"Did the psych tell you this?" I asked. Laurie, the psych from the interpersonal therapy clinic, had started counseling Bobby when the two employees from BJV joined Bill's law firm. Her fees, one hundred and fifty loonies per session, were payable post-settlement. The number of sessions had intensified lately to three times a week; today's had lasted two hours in the afternoon.

Bobby didn't answer. He knew, as did I, that he wasn't a loony, just a brain-injured, disabled doctor. The counseling sessions he was forced to endure—on the heels of the repeated neuropsych tests that had made him sick—had a purpose. They had a good grip on him and were using the sessions to twist the screws of misery and mind control, one turn at a time.

49

BURN

IT SEEMED I HAD CREATED A CONCERN IN THE CONSORTIUM—for both the plaintiff and the defense lawyers, now fused into one, or so it seemed—by dismissing Allen in November. I'd been forced to hire Allen to write an affidavit to deal with the one that the private investigator had brought to my office. Meanwhile, Allen's fees mushroomed to twelve times his initial retainer, as he had me cross-examined by the defense lawyers over my diary. Bill sat with the defense team at the cross-examination. There were other faces—law students, I was told. Donald, the appendage lawyer—who now seemed to have turned into an attack dog for the CMPA—had discussed Bobby's case in their law class.

Bill called my office on November 13 at 1:24 p.m: "Why don't you go along (with Allen) and submit your book?" I'd do no such thing. That would simply exacerbate the scale of harassment, now and in the future. I'd learned a valuable lesson from the last go-around, that lawyers demand everything under the sun: "There shouldn't be any secret between the client and the lawyer." However, for the sake of saving lawyer-hours and discovering the hidden agenda, I'd learned to ask precisely what information was needed, for what reason and what he was going to do with it afterwards. I'd also learnt to throw in, "Haven't I given it already? Besides, it was supposed to be a privileged document." They never returned the documents, and often asked for the same ones again.

But Bill knew that I'd have to find another lawyer, as a flurry of

MEDICAL MALADY

documents bearing the case management judge's name in quotation marks, implying that she'd signed them, started flying in from Donald. Apart from attempting to suction out my diary, they had plans that I had no knowledge of at the time, not all of which were designed to harass, humiliate and decimate our family finances. Joan, Bill's secretary from CMPA, found out that I'd had discussions with Virg—one of the lawyers I had contacted when Brian had dropped out of our case—to defend the diary, before Virg was to receive the files from Allen. It became apparent that they all belonged to the same club—the Law Society—where the upcoming mediation was announced to take place. Virg was propped up now—it seemed their playbook called for the step prior to the judge conducting mediation—to legitimize a looming injustice.

Head bent, legs straddling the chair in front, Bobby was catnapping on his couch. He let out a whimper as I walked in. The apartment door was unlocked. No work, nor lack of advice—much of which was adverse and conflicting—burdened Bobby's psyche of late. The advice seemed to be flooding in, not only from the medical jungle but the legal one as well. Funny, Marc's letter on his bed that day read that his father was "his greatest ally." I remembered when I had taken him back to Calgary for his final set of discoveries, Joan had referred to me as his "big bad dad" for refusing to be fleeced further.

Subtlety wasn't one of Bill's attributes. You should talk, peculiarly he would say, raising his voice in frustration and hostility on the blower, with the clockwork of a collection agency. "Where the hell is the dough?" It seemed that every time that I'd visit Bobby those days, Bill would call with the demand—now raised to $400,000 for his so called "war chest" for the fictional trial. I refused to budge, or rather, Gale did, by refusing to mortgage or sell our house. I had already taken up a credit line, having exhausted all available cash. For Bill, the contingency undertaking now conveniently forgotten, $54,000 was not enough. However, drumming up the so-called trial would significantly raise his take from the impending settlement.

There were other harassing calls: a demand for Bobby's tax returns

PART 6: SASKATOON, 1998

since 1991, and for which we'd already been hassled by a different body. The accounting firm who'd examined the returns said in a letter, "It is appalling that Revenue Canada 'reviewed' Bobby's returns for 1995, 1996 and 1997 at such a traumatic time in your life. It appears that they were picking on Bobby through the piece."

THURSDAY, DECEMBER 31, 1998, 8:37 A.M. I FELT A CHILL of arctic wind on my face as I walked across the large parking lot toward the Chinook Mall. I wondered not about the esoteric Y2K hype driving the nation close to the new millennium, but about what would've happened if I'd convinced Gale to mortgage or sell the house for the phony "war chest," or taken the advice that Bobby had passed on: "Why don't you just burn the diary. You won't have to produce it then."

I brought Bobby back to Calgary on a Saturday, for sessions at BJV on Tuesday at 10 A.M. and Wednesday at 11 A.M.. The lawyers, now fused together in my mind, weren't in the business of clarity, but of confusion. I got the troubling transcripts later. They were sniffing for contributory negligence—Bobby's fault—going as far back as 1985. They grilled him on his relationship with me, as if to vaporize any remnants of the family bond that might have remained after countless counseling sessions. The questions were hurled ad nauseam, perhaps to ensure that the victim and his fortification were ready for the JDR, to cut the deal. A subrogate claim for the surrogates—those who help Bobby—was brought up and included, but none involving the family. We were tricked out of existence. Lying in wait was the emerging plot that blindsided me. An all-out war was at our doorstep.

50

HIJACK

THE DECLARATION OF WAR ARRIVED in a three-and-a-half-line email from Bill on January 25, 1999, that read, "I understand that you may be asserting an in-trust claim against your son in respect of the help that you have provided over and above what might be expected of a normal parent . . ."

There were explosives hidden in those words—"claim against your son," "normal parent"—set to detonate.

Four days later, Friday, I was getting ready to leave work to pick up Bobby from his apartment and head for the airport. A missile landed in my inbox: "I will not be able to present anything to the other parties . . . you may have be dealt with at a later time and that it be severed from any resolution of other matters." It made no sense—grammatically or otherwise. What other matters? While Bill's true motive behind sending those emails remained unclear, I could sense the flash before the strike—a harbinger of hell.

I walked into Bobby's apartment. He was ready; I could hear him from the hallway. But the sound of the door opening turned his voice to a whisper; his cell phone slapped closed. Who was it? Oh, it's Helen. Bobby appeared glum; the instructions he'd just received over the telephone didn't click. His brain injury, he confirmed much later, made him vulnerable and easily manipulated.

I WHEELED BOBBY INTO THE RECEPTION AREA of Bill's relocated office on the 6th floor of 555 5th at 11th Ave, as instructed, first thing

PART 6: SASKATOON, 1998

in the morning. I'd taken the week off work to help Bobby to the JDR, to check his blood sugar, to administer insulin and antiseizure medications, to give him lunch and to be at the meeting.

An ambush waited in the spacious hall. Bill marched right up to me, eyeballs to eyeballs, and barked like a hostile guard that tolerated no intrusion.

"Now leave," he said. He wanted nothing to do with the alien I had become, trash in the way of the pot of gold.

"What about . . ." I pointed to the envelope I'd been asked to produce for the JDR.

"We'll deal with that later." He snatched the envelope and kept pushing forward, until we were nearly butting heads. I stepped backward to avoid falling, until my back was nearly against the door.

"What about Bobby?" I asked, stalling.

"I put you on notice: there would be no mediation if you showed up anywhere within the perimeter of the Law Society building. Now get the hell out," he snarled.

Jamie came out of his office across the hall and leaned against the door frame to witness the commotion. Bobby sat in his wheelchair in stunned silence. He had never seen me so utterly powerless and humiliated before. He hadn't seen Gale and me robbed of our dignity in the hospitals during or following his coma.

The door slammed as I went out. I took the elevator down to the street. I felt that we were being held hostage by a lawyer from hell, backed up by an army of defendants with unlimited resources. Hijacked, Bobby had no choice but to obey. I had no choice but to leave, or Bobby would see no settlement from the lawsuit we'd been fighting since his poisoning and injuries. Joan brought Bobby home that night—a broken, frightened soul.

THE LAW SOCIETY AUDITORIUM, February 1, 1999, was a beehive of activity. Bill assembled his team: his junior, Jamie; Pat (University of Montreal law department); Trev (his new-hire co-counsel, to replace Marc); and last, the subservient plaintiff. Bobby was brain injured and washed out, dredged from yet another bout of hospitalization. He was expendable to the doctors, a bridge to the loot for the lawyers, worn down by the torture of neuropsych tests, numerous psych counseling sessions, and medications—which if held back or delayed would disorient, impair judgment or precipitate seizures and bring him to his knees. The brilliant first born, whose ambition in life was to be a neurologist, had been inflated by the horde, but was now alone in the arena. Simply holding back the rest periods that allowed him to focus and function would advantage the defendants.

The defense lead lawyers—Mart (CMPA), Ken (JGH), and Louise (FHH)—faced Bill's team around the oval conference table of the consortium, the inner circle linked through the Law Society, by the lawyers and for the lawyers. There were the subservients to the CMPA lead—Don (Panis) and Roon (Jen). The remaining twenty-one lawyers sat on benches on the far side of the room and watched the show.

The omnipotent ICU doc wasn't there; he'd gone the way of many of his patients. Scho reportedly was there, representing the doctors.

The Chinese restaurant, through its insurance company, had tabled a million; I'd read the letter of January 21. JGH apparently made overtures to match. The mediation was mainly about CMPA and FHH. Roon wasn't on the distribution list for the defendant's damage report, indicating that Jen would walk. Panis had been the puny player, unworthy in the lawsuit, except perhaps for the services of his lawyer, who had as it appeared assumed the role of an attack dog that kept the family out of the mediation by dirty tricks. The mediation wasn't about going to trial—it was about portioning the damage and liability between the parties representing the defense. But the talk of the trial apparently had a twin purpose: in addition to raising the lawyer's take, it was designed to drain away the family finances, so that we couldn't fight back, now or in the future.

The only lawyer who wasn't allowed in was Virg's junior, Grub. He wanted a retainer, which I'd declined, but he went anyway. Bill told him to treat Bobby and his family as adversaries, a fact that Grub documented in a circuitous letter. The CMPA denied him entry.

51

CHILL

SATURDAY, FEBRUARY 6, 7:45 A.M. BREAKFAST WAS SERVED. A bowl of oatmeal, raisins and sliced banana—a spicy concoction Gale prepared from scratch that Bobby had become fond of—and coffee that he liked, cooled down with plenty of milk. He preferred slurping from his cup without lifting it, before his meds fully kicked in. He liked the table enough to have had us buy one just like it for him, in Montreal before Day Zero. Despite all the attempts to revise history in his mind, he kept having flashbacks, more readily at times.

"Funny," Bobby quipped. "Jen's lawyer cried out to the judge the first day: 'Why am I here; my client is innocent.' Bill snapped back: 'Your client may have tried to kill mine!'"

"He got that right," I said, as I started to inject his belly with twin insulin shots.

The JDR broke off after merely two days of negotiation—a known CMPA tactic—until Bobby had gotten the word the previous night that they would meet again in the morning. The judge would be flown in from Victoria for the case he'd reportedly dubbed "Peanut Justice."

"He is here," Gale hollered from the bay window, through the blooming hibiscus.

"Hurry up, will you," Bobby rushed me.

"Don't you want him to see me inject you?"

"Nope." We were enemies in their eyes.

The doorbell rang. Gale let Trev, the new co-counsel, come in and offered him one of the round stools to sit on. He was tall, handsome, and stingy with words, but sat patiently while Bobby finished his breakfast. He'd never handled a wheelchair before, it seemed, nor had he practiced law for long. I helped Bobby to the car while Trev put the wheelchair into the trunk. They took off, as did my thoughts, to the Law Society auditorium.

THE LULL IN THE JDR OPENED THE WINDOW for us to witness the lopsided machinations through Bobby's eyes and ears, and his myoclonic childlike sketches. I could imagine the judge sitting by the blackboard on the first day, reading the defense counsel's brief, listening to their absurd presentations, yet maintaining a straight face. Was he thinking, as I did, that the medical experts who'd claimed that a foreign object lodged in the lung—and on suction for nearly two hours—did not cause obstruction, thus hypoxia, should be allowed to experience it themselves? They'd be in a hurry to change their minds, unless, of course, they lacked the most basic understanding of physiology and fluid flow, made handsome profits by rendering tainted medical opinion, or owed the CMPA big time, or all of the above. One of the doctors, an intensivist, profited from both sides, first from the family when I paid, and later from the defense, who'd probably poached him in desperation.

The CMPA couldn't seem to find an expert save one schooled in gynecology–radiology–orthopedics, and another schooled in apartheid South Africa, whose fifty years of practice allowed him to make this profound pronouncement: "It is not clear when the nasogastric tube was inserted or who inserted it. It's quite possible, since it is a common procedure, that it was a non-medical person." He went on to opine, " . . . the iatrogenic factor applies only to Dr. Bobby. . . .." In other words, the victim was to blame for inserting the tube in his lung and putting it on suction, while he was thrashing around and collapsed in a coma.

The second day of the JDR was reportedly set aside for the discussion of damages, and queries from the mediator, who by now had befriended Bobby. Roon, as it turned out, didn't turn up. He walked,

PART 6: SASKATOON, 1998

and therefore Jen walked, scot-free, but certainly not guilt-free or free from suspicion. The ER doctors weren't turned in for misleading and apparent falsification of charts—supposedly a felony—and one that endangered a patient's life, biased further treatment and caused permanent disability.

JGH apparently matched the Chinese restaurant, who reportedly raised their portion; CMPA was said to put a pittance on the table but improved as the day wore on. The $20 million-lawsuit was whittled down, reportedly by the defense's citing of contributory negligence, using incredible defense-expert reports that blamed Bobby. FHH came forth with a pittance, and the money on the table with the other two defendants totaled nearly $3-1/2 million. The voluminous reports on the long-term functional needs and cost analysis, assessment of loss of income and future cost of care, multi-disciplinary consensus opinions on future care needs and cost analysis all seemed farcical. It was window dressing that had caused physical and mental torture for the victim.

"They have the gall to table this letter from a psychiatrist," Bobby said, "to reduce the settlement amount." He was upset. The page displayed the letterhead of the Rocky View Hospital in Calgary, which claimed to have offered him a psychiatry position. The structured settlement offered, he said, was miniscule, and designed to push him into the arms of the lawyer. I listened as I helped Neilly with his engineering school application; he didn't want any part of a career in medicine or law, although he was just as talented as his doctor siblings were. I didn't hold that against him; on the contrary, I'd rather see him make an honest living.

There's a lot to be cleaned up in the self-regulated professions and the CMPA. It has become a bonanza for lawyers, who seemed to have traded honesty for dirty tricks. It costs taxpayers immensely at the expense of the standard of care, although technology has made it possible to raise it and reduce Medicare costs. Ours didn't appear to be an isolated case.

BLURRY-EYED AND EXHAUSTED, Bobby called me at 5:42 P.M.

"I am about to go and sign the documents (of settlement)."

"Who is there with you?"

"No one. They are going to La Chaumiere for dinner after." Bobby had more things to add but it was pointless, I thought. The peril wouldn't end with the pot of gold; they'd find words to shackle this hostage. Nevertheless, he was pumped up—by the family of lawyers and the judge—ready to be taken away into the wilderness and devoured. The remnants from the domino of wrongdoings would be downloaded to the scavengers, and whatever happened to him would be forgotten, leaving me with the burden of memory.

The next day, I wheeled him to the 12:15 P.M. Air Canada flight to Toronto, as I'd done time and again. An eerie silence beset him. There was no joy at settling the lawsuit, but rather a feeling of being herded into a ruinous tunnel.

"Aren't you happy?" I asked, trying to break the ice, knowing that the lawyers and their significant others had celebrated their victory late last night; they had reasons to.

"I am still disabled," he said.

"We are looking for a house in Toronto, thinking of a condo downtown for you and for us."

"Not for me. I have to go as far away from my parents as possible."

"Is that the deal?"

There was a wall of silence as we waited on the tarmac. I introduced Bobby to Kelly, one of my colleagues, at the counter by the gate. He was on the plane in the next seat.

"What about the girl who seemed to have a lot to hide in Montreal? And the doctors who'd apparently falsified the charts? What about turning the files over to the authorities?"

"I have to move on; it's up to you now."

Bobby seemed worried about the "deal." Fear was etched on his face. Had he been threatened, the way I had been ambushed? That wouldn't be a surprise. He was brutally frank otherwise, recalling that Bill and his girlfriend had dropped him off at Oakfern after their late night

PART 6: SASKATOON, 1998

celebration. Bobby had napped nearby in his wheelchair. He asked Bill on the ride back, "What about the money my parents spent?"

"We don't pay."

"What if he writes a book?"

"He might; he is driven." Laughter. "He'd slam me if he did."

The plane landed in daylight at Pearson Airport. A chill was in the air as we got off. Bobby broke the news as I looked for the luggage: Helen would be waiting at the arrival gate; I wouldn't have to take him to his apartment, not anymore. I dragged his large blue suitcase off the conveyor belt. It felt enormously heavy, filled with everything that we hadn't already moved from our Calgary home to his apartment. He knew that would be his last visit home, a marching order imposed on him—an elaborate scheme devised well in advance, perhaps detailed in their operating manual and lectured in workshops and seminars.

Helen was waiting outside the gate. She grabbed the handle of the suitcase out of my hand and tugged it away as fast as she could. Bobby peddled his wheelchair with his feet, following her like an obedient boy. I watched them both disappear through the entrance of the parking garage across the slow airport traffic that stopped just to let them pass. There was no goodbye.

PART 7:
PITTSBURGH, 2000

52

DEEP END

NOVEMBER 2000. BOBBY WAS GOING INTO THE DEEP END of the pool without his lifejacket. Outside, behind the steamy glass walls of the Eau Claire Y, our eyes caught him in horror. Gale screamed, and I watched in panic, but there was no one to hear. We couldn't stop him from drowning.

It was only a dream—one that woke me up in a cold afternoon sweat—but the lifejacket, or lack of it, was real. The crooks had cast him adrift and separated him from the family that had kept him alive and afloat for the last six years.

I must have fallen asleep after coming back from work. I got out of bed, grabbed my gym bag and went out the door. I waited by the window of the elevator bay on the 8th floor. The sun setting into the cradle of the green hills over the river valley, like Valium, settled my mind and moved my thoughts in a direction that seemed fitting at this stage of my career and our lives. The Oxford apartments in the Monroeville suburb of Pittsburgh were next to a gigantic racquet club we frequented. It preserved our hearts and sanity. Living here was a seismic change, but one that gave me time to regroup and recover, and, most importantly, to reflect.

At Foothills in Calgary, a neuro-nurse had once told me the story of a ninety-year-old man in the ICU: "I buried four wives in my life, but burying my sixty-year-old son was the hardest," he said. Perhaps that explained why we couldn't forget what we had gone through with our first born. The medical–legal system seemed to want us to forget

PART 7: PITTSBURGH, 2000

him, and him us: get out of his life to keep the medical–legal malpractice a secret. Amazing to what extent they had gone to guarantee it, as we discovered later.

Shortly after Bobby and Helen had left me at the arrival terminal, Gale, Neilly and I went to see Bobby in his apartment. Helen was sitting on the couch, looking at a church newsletter on her lap, a motionless pencil between her fingers. Bobby had a cold; he was wheezy. The apartment was filthy. Bellwoods had stopped government-sponsored services. Now that he had money, apparently they had said he could pay for it privately—forcing him squarely into the hands of the surrogate mother, the boys and others that had surfaced through the medical–legal woodwork. They provided services that he could've gotten from his family for free; we'd moved to Toronto by then. He said he was being hit with subrogated claims from the governments for the healthcare services they'd provided since his poisoning and iatrogenic injuries. Bobby found himself sick, confused and alone.

He lifted his head from his chest and said to me, "You may come after me as well, like all the others. Go ahead, sue me. You would lose; you won't get a penny." It was painful to see and hear him like this, more so to sense that he had been manipulated to be distrustful of his own family. He had probably been told that the family of lawyers would fight for him. They would cheer him on to ruin and collect their fees in glee.

"We won't; we don't want your money," I said. "If we got our expenses back, over $300,000, we would've bought a condo for you in Toronto; this seems to be an ideal time." I'd brought brochures to show him prior to the JDR; perhaps they were still displayed in the corner of his apartment by the kitchen. But he'd hear none of it.

"Now go—leave," he said, mimicking Bill. One other time, the building superintendent had turned us away from the entrance. "He is a very private man; he doesn't want to be disturbed." Someone had told the super of the contrived dispute with his family. Telephone and emails were intercepted and screened. We became strangers—worse, enemies—overnight.

MEDICAL MALADY

I recalled when I'd gone to Virg's office to pick up the diary fragments that the case management judge had ordered me to produce for her exclusive examination. I'd had a nasty feeling then that the system was setting us up for a legal fight with Bobby if we wanted to get all the family's expenses back. Grub had broached the subject at the time, but I would hear none of it. Yet word spreads fast in the small community of medical malpractice lawyers in Calgary. Bobby was probably told about it to make him angry at me, perhaps even before Grub had presented me with the idea. I couldn't imagine, despite all the advance warnings from the very early days, that the powerful and mighty would be so vindictive against ones so vulnerable in the society—the victims of iatrogenic injuries.

A check arrived in the mail from the lawyers for a meager $3000. I refused to accept it, and returned it promptly. I asked them to send it back to where it came from, and demanded to see a copy of the letter that accompanied it. As I suspected, it seemed crafted to mislead. The letter was from Mart: "This money is sent to you in trust that it not be disbursed until you have sent to me confirmation of receipt of this amount and confirmation that receipt of the total amount due of $6,331 is accepted by your client . . . in full satisfaction of all claims, including cost claims." Grub had no authority to sign such a letter or accept the check. Shortly after I returned the check, an unsigned letter arrived from the law firm in which Virg and Grub had been partners, advising me that the money I'd refused to accept had been sent to the Law Society. I concluded that the Law Society appears to have profited from the wrongdoings. Virg, I was told, worked for them, which is why she wouldn't file a complaint to the Law Society on our behalf.

The sun went down for the day. The elevator on the 8th floor must have come up and down a few times by the time I was snapped back into our modest existence in Pittsburgh by the noise of the neighbor—a Pittsburgh Steelers football player—on his way to the gym. I went down to the ground level, walked left across the long parking lot decorated with dogwood trees, climbed up the stairs and entered the

PART 7: PITTSBURGH, 2000

club through the terrace entrance, thinking that to forget would be to help them keep the secret.

"Haven't seen you before." An abrupt interruption came from a locker, kitty corner from mine. The man looked dignified, fifty something, white-haired, about to put his racquet away. People were friendly in western Pennsylvania, not prodding. But he was. He asked me what I did, where I worked, and where I was from. I returned the favor. "And you?"

"I am an attorney." A proud response from one expecting reverence. A flash fire crossed my face. The words, "A fucking lawyer!" shot out of my vocal cords.

He was taken aback. I apologized profusely for the spontaneous combustion. He didn't wait around. He picked up his towels and hurried his bare essentials to the showers.

I WENT TO WORK THE NEXT MORNING AMID AZALEA BUSHES in blazing bloom. An anomaly in chemical land? I pondered. My mind wasn't on the analysis of the night-shift data on my desk, but on the people around me. Our executive vice-president had colon cancer; he came to work with a $5000 precision micro-injector pump in a pouch that carried out post-radiation chemotherapy while he worked. My best operator had had part of his cheekbone removed for cancer, his eyes bulged out and his voice was nasal; you needed to pay closer attention to his utterances to communicate. Our human resources manager had ovarian cancer and couldn't bear the children she dearly loved; one of the other operators had suffered a stroke. Our plump president—who drank three pints of beer at lunch—wouldn't agree to send flowers to the hospital until he died. He didn't, and he came back to work. Yet, they all seemed happy. Anomaly indeed. They would be history in Montreal or Calgary, I thought.

It didn't take long to figure out the healthcare system in this city of a million people, devastated by the demise of steel. It had six large hospitals, three MRI machines in each. Our secretary had an MRI of her knee within a week of requesting one. I recalled that Bobby hadn't

MEDICAL MALADY

been able to get one when he needed it, shortly after Day Zero. If he had, he wouldn't have been left to die of the devastating diagnosis. Here, the emphasis was on diagnostic precision and aggressive treatment, on putting workers back to work, to keep the richest economy in the world humming. We were given health insurance in return, and a premise that they'd treat you until they could treat no more. That's what preserved the knowledge workers, who in turn preserved the workplace—a symbiotic relationship.

I'd wanted to leave the dark side of socialized medicine behind when I decided to move to western Pennsylvania. Now I realized that I needed to leave to tell the rest of our story—the story of the abuse of the most vulnerable in the society by the most powerful—or it would die. The time arrived in June 2001. Our tiny Toyota was full to the rearview mirror. I closed the apartment, wrote a note on a ripped corner of the Pittsburgh Post Gazette, and slipped it under the building manager Juanita's door. The William Penn highway to the Pennsylvania Turnpike north wound like a serpent hugging the Allegheny Mountains. I thought of dropping by the old research center at the New Kensington exit—just over the Allegheny River Bridge. Instead, I picked up the desolate Interstate 79 to Erie, to the Greater Toronto Area. I'd balance my time between preparing for my next assignment and breaking through the barriers that had been raised around Bobby.

TUESDAY, SEPTEMBER 11, 2001. IN A STRANGE TWIST OF FATE, I ended up in Winnipeg—instead of my destination—Fort McMurray—on the morning of the terrorist attack on New York. The captain on the Air Canada 8:40 A.M. non-stop flight from Toronto to Edmonton made an announcement: "FAA is shutting down all airports in the US of A." He made an emergency landing, as did twenty-one other planes. Pandemonium in the airport. The oil company I was to visit found a hotel room in downtown Winnipeg. There was no way out of the city for four days. In a stroke of luck, I met Dr. Seshia in a downtown restaurant the day following the infamy, and we traded our stories of the events that had left permanent scars on our lives.

PART 7: PITTSBURGH, 2000

Apart from all the troubles he'd been through, Seshia didn't get paid all that was due to him when the case settled. He complained to the Law Society. He was told that he should get the money from Bobby's family.

"Did you know we didn't receive a penny from the settlement?" I said, surprised.

The man couldn't be trusted, he said.

"That goes for the horde, the fraternity of the medical–legal system."

"He had the gall to ask me for an opinion on another case!"

"Have you had any contact with the Quebec City lawyer?"

"He called me up for a case. His client didn't have any money, wanted my opinion for free."

At the time, some of the CMPA lawyers billed $1000 an hour, apparently. Who was to keep track of their hours? There were twenty-one lawyers of various stripes involved in our case. Victims, on the contrary, lost a capable and compassionate witness.

53

SWITCH

SATURDAY, FEBRUARY 8, 2003. RADIO AM 680 blares the traffic and weather report confirming the cold yet sunny salt-coated road past Kingston. Gale looks out the window and gives a sigh of relief. We'd been held up on this stretch of Hwy 416 in snow before, in the dead of winter. She doesn't fancy delay; certainly not now—she wants to see Mon. She pictures her as her little girl on one hand and on the other, a grown woman, a confident no-nonsense doctor preparing for her exams: Royal College and a black belt in karate. Mon keeps her distance, avoids talking about the lawsuit or any other matter related to it that has engulfed our lives since Bobby's poisoning and iatrogenic injuries. It isn't often that she calls for help.

"What did she say? I turn down the volume to ask."

"Her exam is this week, fellowship exam in May," she retorts. "She has no time to look after him."

Bobby flies in from Thunder Bay at just about the same time we drive to Ottawa. His colleagues have loaned him the money to pay for his psychiatry review course, also this week at the Royal Ottawa Hospital, prior to his fellowship exam in April. He wants to stay with Mon for the duration, but she isn't prepared to be his attendant. She needs time to prepare for her final exam, the distillation of five years of training to be a specialist; karate is her stress relief.

ALL GOES WELL IN THE SPACIOUS HIGH-RISE APARTMENT UNTIL Sunday afternoon: Bobby has lunch, goes to sleep on the living room

PART 7: PITTSBURGH, 2000

futon that turns into an elegant sofa. A couple of hours go by. He gets up, and, as sick as he appears, manages to drag himself to the bathroom and empty his bloated gut into the sink. The sink promptly plugs with chunks of undigested food particles and other slimy substances. Thankfully, the superintendent of the urban building complex is around. The thirty-year-old drainpipe ruptures in the unplugging process, and vomitus comes flooding down the cupboard below—rendering the toilet paper rolls, Kleenex boxes and such utterly soggy.

Mon says, "Well . . . I have to go do the groceries." She promptly goes out, slamming the door behind. Gale follows her to the elevator, leaving me to care for the passed-out grown-up on the sofa, and to clean up the area; the maintenance crew won't work on a slippery floor. I struggle for three hours before the apartment is livable again, just in time for the groceries to arrive. Things could have been worse, I console myself, not knowing what's coming next.

The following morning, Mon drives Bobby to his course on her way to work at the Civic Hospital. He doesn't take his wheelchair but walks, to and from the car, presumably to assure himself and us that he is indeed in control, and registers for the course. "I may look like a patient," he says to the receptionist at the lobby, before entering the auditorium, "but I am a psychiatrist taking the review course."

Bobby returns to the apartment in the afternoon by cab. His insulin needle broke at lunch. He decides to take another shot at home, on his own, to his belly. His vision seems as cloudy as the vial, and he has difficulty putting the cap back on the fine needle. He puts it away finally, and, moments later, he is deep in sleep.

Soon it's dark. Gale remembers that he'd made a dinner engagement with Supriya, the medical resident friend from Calgary—now a divorcée in Ottawa. She hollers out at the top of her lungs. He gets up when the hollering gets intense, but is unable to move. His stomach churns, squeezing the remains up his gullet and onto the pillow and sofa, elegant no more. He could've drowned in his vomit if we weren't here, I thought. Stomach empty, he hobbles to the bathroom, and we wait. The door finally opens. Out comes a man, unrecognizable. He is slower than a geriatric sloth, drags himself to the kitchen chair, and sits frozen in a stupor with his head immobile and heavy on the bare wooden table. Gale and the two docs—Mon and Supriya—help him to the Ottawa General, where he is diagnosed as having seizures with no visible signs. They return from the hospital, with Bobby, in the wee hours of the morning. He spends the day sleeping; we spend it wondering.

PITTSBURGH HAD GIVEN US A FRESH START, but no handle to knock down the barriers erected around Bobby. Unexpectedly, a break came in January, when he called at 6:30 A.M. to say that he had arrived on a red-eye flight from Calgary. We had wondered where he was on his birthday, Christmas, and New Year's Day. Bill had been throwing lavish parties for each of the past four years since the JDR, Bobby said. Fewer of the roster of friends—names we had been asked to provide as witnesses for the fictitious trial—attend, but a growing number of Bill's family members do. In a voice more melancholic than myoclonic, he announces that he is leaving Toronto, permanently, giving up his apartment, and giving away some of his belongings to the people who insulated him from us.

The conversation ended as abruptly as it began. Gale and I venture out to his apartment, cognizant of the locked door, of the lecture from the building superintendent.

His telephone was disconnected and the building entrance couldn't be opened remotely. Gale called the superintendent. "The moving truck came yesterday," he responded. "He has left!"

"No, he is there," Gale pleaded. "Only his furniture left." The superintendent went to verify, and then walked to the foyer with a woman caretaker and opened the glass door. We began our ascent to the 10th floor, unsure of who or what we'd find.

The door was open. Bobby was sleeping on the bedroom floor, his bare body hugging the same green K-Mart mat that had so often been my makeshift bed prior to the JDR. Now his bedroom was bare, covered with debris from the furniture and belongings that had been there and gone. The other room was cluttered with boxes.

PART 7: PITTSBURGH, 2000

The paintings weren't crated but were left for someone—perhaps the same someone who'd picked up the telephone when we'd called one day, and shouted, "They are after your money again. Do you want to talk?" He seemed exhausted from the red-eye trip; he didn't get up or utter a word.

We left to return later. Neilly and his luggage had to be dropped off at Beck Hall at the University of Waterloo; he was to start his 3rd-year academic term in Engineering. I rushed home to Mississauga to pick up Gale, rushed back to Bobby's apartment in Toronto to see him off, and perhaps, just perhaps, unravel the tangled skein. He'd advised Gale earlier on the telephone not to come, but we couldn't stay away. He was to catch the 8:45 P.M. Tango airline flight to Thunder Bay. We got to the apartment late. Without keys to the front entrance, we waited, biting nails, until someone let us in. We went up and knocked. The radio was blaring. Between gaps in music, we could hear his signature snore, inviting us to knock louder, in unison.

"Come, the door is open," he responded groggily.

"No, it isn't."

He got up from the decrepit black swivel chair in the living room to open the door and wobbled back to doze, through the paper strewn around the floor, and the boxes, some full, some empty. His black travel bags were at different stages of preparedness. The adjacent room was empty but dirty; the vacuum cleaner that I'd helped him buy when I moved him to the apartment in 1996 was still in the closet but in a state of disrepair.

"We thought you had help."

"Ana came and picked up the box full of drinks at four. She had to attend to some business."

"What about the lesbian couple?"

"They came in the afternoon, but didn't stay round. They had to leave."

Bobby appeared like a derelict, his face full of beard and topped with disheveled, thinning hair. It was obvious he hadn't had anything to eat; he was shaking.

MEDICAL MALADY

Gale began to cry. "How can I help? I feel so helpless."

Bobby's so-called friends and employees were all gone, and so was all his money. One of the lesbian couple, who had worked in a bank, took him to the CIBC bank for a loan. He owed the bank $150,000, he said. The other, who had apparently worked at the Ministry of Health, got him a shredder and helped shred his documents, which they used in packing. We followed him to the airport terminal, the same one at which he'd left me bewildered the day after his settlement. He was leaving us now, again, to "go as far away from his parents as possible," to his exile.

HERE IN OTTAWA, A MONTH HAS GONE BY SINCE WE SAW him at the LPH in Thunder Bay. His memory—of the poisoning and iatrogenic injuries—has been revised in his mind, but there have been no symptoms like the kind we see now. He lies motionless, motion sick at times, as if the futon is a rickety boat in some stormy sea. Gale covers her mouth with both her hands, and Mon bolts to her bedroom as Bobby throws up again in the afternoon. His dense black beard and hairy chest are smeared with the bile ejected from his empty stomach. The psych review course on Forensic Psychiatry, Mental Retardation, and Anorexia Nervosa and Bulimia in Ottawa General goes on without one of the paid participants, as the three of us observe and argue over his future. He has been getting sicker in Thunder Bay.

Bobby musters enough strength on Wednesday, February 12, 2003, to get up and go to the final day of the psych review course. Mon and Gale drop him off at the door, no wheelchair, and he falls on the way in. A passerby gives Mon a hand to lift his sluggish body from the sidewalk. Once inside, he waves them off and hauls himself to the auditorium along with nearly two hundred other psychiatrists attending the review course to be licensed to practice in Canada. Some of them have completed their residency requirements, as Bobby has, and are qualified to practice in Ontario on a limited license. Bobby attends two hours of the session until the coffee break, and then asks for a bed to lie down. There is no bed in the first-floor foyer. Boni, the secretary,

PART 7: PITTSBURGH, 2000

sits with him on a bench outside the auditorium when he throws up again, disoriented. The course director sends him to the Ottawa Civic ER by ambulance.

We arrive at the ER within an hour of receiving the message. At our suggestion, they call a neurologist. A young neurologist responds, and soon becomes overwhelmed by the many complications and medications. He suggests that a medicine specialist see him as well. The specialist in turn decides to transfer him to the Ottawa General neuro observation unit by ambulance.

The next day, I get an unexpected telephone call—a plea, in fact—from the hospital. Would you come to sign a form? Gale had been visiting Bobby in the ward with Mon. I ask her to meet me at the admitting office and rush to the hospital. She rummages through Bobby's wallet pouch while we wait for our turn on the main floor. His Liberty Health card expires in a couple of days and he is not on the LPH payroll. The hospital wants me to sign the admitting form and be responsible for the costs. As if these issues aren't enough of a surprise, Gale stumbles on to another one. My jaw drops when she cries out, "Where on earth are the Gabapentin capsules in the dossette?"

"What the . . . look at all these Lipidil capsules!"

In each of the six chambers of the medicine dispenser—prepared back at LPH in Thunder Bay for the eight-day trip to Ottawa—the Gabapentin *antiseizure medication* capsules are absent. In their place are Lipidil, which are *cholesterol lowering* capsules. Since his arrival, Bobby has been completely deprived of one and overdosed with the other. Bingo! The source of the convulsions, disorientation, and unsteadiness—symptoms similar to that reported occasionally by some of the staff at LPH immediately following our visit to Thunder Bay in January—becomes obvious. We waste no time in letting it be known; not knowing whether the deadly game is an honest mistake or being played for a purpose.

Gale and I ask to meet with a staff doctor. We get Andrew, a neurology resident, instead. He brings up the issue of Bobby's poor relations with his family, me in particular. The focus on the family relations—concocted or not—shifts the spotlight away from the drug switch. Someone has briefed Andrew on our right to be concerned. Gale had discovered something else as well—a check made out to Bill for nearly $1500, before Bobby left Thunder Bay.

Saturday, February 15, 2003. The medications reinstated, Bobby's breathing improves like the flick of a switch; he isn't nauseous anymore, his energy level takes a dramatic upsurge. The episode also exposes a piece of paper that appointed Bill, now Queen's Counsel, as Bobby's Estate Trustee. It states: "I give all my real property and all my personal property, (including all property over which I may have a general power of appointment), regardless of where it is located, to my trustee . . ." The document goes on to state that visitation is open, however, and that medical care is decided by POA—power of attorney, personal care in consultation with the medical staff—clearing the way to the bucket.

54

TRIPLE PLAY

"I AM IN THE COMPANY OF A BEAUTIFUL WOMAN," Bobby calls.

"Who's there with you?" I ask.

"None of your business," he responds in this moment of pride. I hear her giggling in the background. It must be Karen, one of his classmates, on locum in Thunder Bay. Bobby sounds upbeat. He has gone back to that northern city. LPH has put him on payroll, given him drug insurance and his life back—a life that was nearly taken away, yet again. The drug switch is hushed, but for the paper trail left in its wake.

The Ottawa story, however—still fresh in his mind—has driven him out of the fortress of secrecy built around him by the lawyers and the psychologists, sociologists and psychiatrists. He has moved from the dreary psych residence into a place of his own. There, at last, the curtain of fog lifts, taking with it swirling particulates of misinformation that had been planted in his mind.

A FULL CIRCLE WE SEEM TO HAVE COME—from the day after the JDR to this day—as Gale and I pick him up from Gate D of the arrival deck at the Toronto airport, the same spot he wheeled away from, with Helen, without saying goodbye. "Does this gate remind you of anything?" I ask.

It doesn't. His memory may be wiped clean or distorted, but the moment is still vivid in my mind. He was like a programmed robot, following instructions: "Go as far away from your parents as possible."

"When do you think you really came to your senses, after the coma?" I ask, passing a galaxy of streetlights pitching shadows on our faces.

"Things are coming together only for the last couple of years," says Bobby, buckled in and relaxed in the back seat. Something sets my mind adrift to the day he set out on his goodbye trip from Jen. He had spoken just as clearly and convincingly today as he had then.

I move to the HOV[25] lane, past the Mississauga skyline that has matured since Bobby was exiled north. Alert and awake as we arrive home, he walks up the stairs to the kitchen and announces, "I'm hungry. What do you have?" A scurrying rabbit triggers the floodlight in the backyard, illuminating the naked vine, as we play a game of Scrabble after dinner. It is just like the old times—he scores over 200; Gale and I, merely 150 each.

"How do you rationalize this score and the disappearance of your money?" I ask, half joking.

"Some areas of the brain don't come back as fast as others."

"Some may think your residency training isn't . . ."

"Not at all; my medical knowledge came back first. The rest is a gradual process," he interrupts.

"You think people took advantage of you?"

"Yes . . . neuropsych tests don't tell everything."

"The reason the defense needed mind manipulators." I am reminded of the Toronto psychologist, who'd entered the scene shortly before the JDR and never took his family history nor showed interest in his background.

"Were you mad at her?"

"Yes, I didn't pay her for the last month; made her life miserable."

"Oh . . . how much?"

"About $1500. I left her a note: 'See you in small claims court.'"

THE SETTLEMENT PAPERS TAKE US BACK to Saturday, February 6, 1999. Exhausted and confused, Bobby called me at 5:42 P.M. and went to sign the handwritten mediation agreement, incomprehensible in his coma-induced fog, to settle *Bobby v. 2625-7949 Quebec, et*

PART 7: PITTSBURGH, 2000

al. Alberta Queens Bench action #9501-09663. Mart and Louise were there to co-sign, and the mediating judge to witness. Other defendants signed on later, but collectively committed to pay the settlement amount of $3,275,000 in trust to Bill by February 19, 1999. On Wednesday evening, Jamie arrived in Toronto with a check in one hand for $1,521,665.42, and in the other an armload of releases. The Nesbitt Burns offices were closed by then, so a hotel, restaurant and entertainment kept James occupied until morning. He took Bobby to JC, an advisor with Nesbitt, and handed over the check. On Friday, he visited JC alone before returning to Calgary.

The releases authorized Bill to withhold an unspecified portion of the settlement money—a hook to hold Bobby hostage and away from his family. The false hope of recovering that money seemed to have forced Bobby to attend Bill's lavish Christmas parties for the four consecutive years, especially when the money that was given to Bobby, in JC's custody, vanished within the first nine months. To separate us from Bobby was to ensure disappearance of the money, and to hide the accounting and distribution of the entire settlement.

"How did you lose all that settlement money in such short order?" I'd asked before he left Thunder Bay. Patty, the accountant that JC had introduced him to sent us statements that told only a part of the convoluted rip-off. Money started disappearing from JC's custody almost immediately, paid out under "Client Request" in large chunks: February 26, $180,960; March 31, $159,442; week of December 1, 2000, $159,840, and numerous smaller chunks. A note, *"Client request is noted where the payee details could not be determined from the records provided,"* was also in the file. Some of the recipients of the smaller chunks were the attendees of Bill's Christmas party and their connections. By March 2000, barely a year after JDR, the looting was nearly complete.

I asked, "Do you know all these people under client request, their individual cuts, besides the ones we recognize?"

A vacant look. I didn't think he knew. His splurging on paintings doesn't explain the loss. The knick-knacks and display-swords came long before the settlement was on the horizon. The cancelled checks, half of which were written by one of the lesbian couple, apparently introduced to him through the MOH, were shredded by her, along with other documents, and used as packaging material for his move to the city of the north.

"First, we were misinformed by the girl, then by the doctors and the hospitals, then by the lawyer, and now by the fair-weather crowd that came out of the medical–legal woodwork." That is spreading wrong-doings far and wide. The one who had started the fire that burned the house down to the ground now melted away, lost in the fraternity.

"Okay, gloat if you like."

There is no gloating here, but on the opposite side of medical maladies, they called it a "triple play." That seems to be the medical–legal malpractice played by the book, from poisoning on Day Zero, to the year following the settlement when the victim's money was all but squandered away, patient supports marginalized and vilified, adverse witnesses punished. The perpetrators remain behind the fortress of secrecy, victimizing the victims over and over and over again.

55

EPILOGUE

TORONTO 2006. SUMMERS COME AND SUMMERS DON'T WAIT. The vines bear witness to them, and oodles more as the years pass. Gale painstakingly stuffs and rolls fifty-five blanched leaves for treats, one after another, and I contemplate the episodes—ahead of the urn—documented in as many chapters.

She wipes her aging brow, hands over the Corelle bowl from the IKEA kitchen table and quips, "What did you say the girl got for her troubles?"

"Plenty." I put the contents in the boiling steamer and wait for the lid to rattle, the whistle to blow. "I've saved this part for last."

THE DEFENDANTS HAD INSURANCE—THE CMPA. We had none. If I am allowed to generalize, patients have no accident insurance against hospital screw-ups or protection from incompetent inexperienced doctors, 50% of whom graduate in the bottom half of their class. Would we drive our car on the road without insurance when the big guys—say the truck drivers—had hit us more than once? They have accident insurance with bottomless coffers, and we live from one paycheck to the next. Almost immediately, the big guys start to discredit, demonize and isolate the victim's only support—his family. If the wrongdoings incapacitate a victim, his family members find themselves alone to face the Goliaths in a legal contest to remedy abhorrent injustices, and lawyers on both sides feast on them.

MEDICAL MALADY

That's how Jen's mother, a busy Calgary psychiatrist, was used during the two-week period in Montreal, when it seemed to me that she was on their payroll. No pangs of conscience appeared to get in her way in slandering the parents of a comatose son, in leaving derogatory and defamatory comments about the patient advocate in the patient's charts, of all places, with the help of a clergy, or blaming the victim for his predicament.

The girl, now a doctor, had been protected in a symbiotic partnership since Day Zero. She didn't just get away with convoluted false statements, but danced away with the reward money wrung out of the settlement. " . . . pay the defendant, *Jen*, the sum of Four Thousand ($4,000.00) for her costs." Early in her career, she appeared to have learned that distortion of facts is rewarded, if the hospitals and the self-regulated, self-serving associations are on side.

WHEN THEY KNOW THE DAMAGE THAT THEY HAVE caused is so deep they can't win, the defendants settle out of court. And they do so grudgingly. Their weapon, wrapped in cold-war secrecy, is to use the victim against his family. The victim—set up to fail—must sign what amounts to a financial self-immolation: " . . . Releasor *Bobby* does hereby agree to indemnify and save harmless the Releasees *the defendants* of and from any and all future claims which may be commenced against the Releasees by or on behalf of the said Releasor or by any other party by way of subrogation or for contribution or indemnity . . ."

The only workable remedy seems to be malpractice insurance for the patients to balance the colossal abuse of power of the CMPA and the lawyers that work for them on both sides.

Malpractice doctors mislead convincingly, and convincingly get away with impunity, right under the nose of all levels of governments. That may be one of the reasons why medicine is called an art and a science; medical ineptitude is pervasive, and unfortunately for the patients, the medical–legal landscape is littered with intellectual dishonesty that ruins the reputation of the majority of diligent doctors

PART 7: PITTSBURGH, 2000

who truly do care, and without whose help Bobby would not be alive today. A conclusion based on a personal account may sound facetious, but it is not far from the reality. No charges were laid against the doctors who apparently falsified Bobby's medical records, seemingly to conceal wrongdoings. The matter was brought to the attention of the medical–legal societies, the provincial and federal governments and the police. Those doctors are still practicing, with one exception: Dr. Spa. The headline in the *Montreal Gazette*, April 28, 1999, read: "MD collapses, dies at inquest . . ."

THE COVER RATTLES. GALE RESPONDS TO THE WHISTLE. "Wasn't the inquest about the one diagonally across from Bobby?" Many summers have blown past since Day Zero, yet it's fresh in our minds what they'd said about the patient she means, though it may not be the one who the inquest was about. "Well, he had a good life; just keep him comfortable—let nature take its course." I was about to step out of the kitchen when Gale reminds me of the written admission of the lead legal sharks of the west: "The case rises and falls with the misplaced nasogastric tube." I meander over to the vines by the rows of Rose of Sharon and think of Ann Lander's wisdom: "The naked truth is always better than the best dressed lie." The Rose of Sharon in full bloom sways in the changing wind.

AUTHOR'S NOTE

The intervening period between completion of this book and today brought many challenges, but none surpassed the trauma of the yesteryears. In case you are wondering, Bobby is now a psychiatrist pursuing many interests: professional, research and academic. Here, in his own words, is how he has been doing of late:

> "Exposing a hidden truth that belies a trusted establishment's promise to "Do no harm" and revealing it to a reading audience who may be unaware of these facts that occur is daunting, yet courageous. A simple medical error transformed my life from a healthy young man to a brain-injured epileptic and insulin-dependent diabetic. Now, 18 years later, fatigue, medications and personal care workers rule part of my life. My ambition, perseverance and determination to do better, recover more, and contribute to medicine continue. Since 1994, I completed my psychiatry residency, completed a subspecialty in community medicine, and taught at a medical school. Now I work with the First Nations with respect to their many problems. I am active physically, with limits, and actively participate as a scholar and a medical researcher. Nothing is ever perfect or easy, but all things considered, what I am currently doing is satisfying."

This book was written from the vantage point of one person, the author. It contains graphic description of events as they unfolded, some of which may be disturbing to some readers. Observations, personal diaries, notes, emails, sketches, photographs, medical records, transcriptions, discovery court documents, telephone conversations and personal communications—recorded or not—were used to write this book and provide a basis for the author's opinions, feelings and inferences.

The purpose of this book is to inform and to form an understanding of medical malady, the existence of which cannot be denied. To think that it will never happen to you is unwise. The book is not intended to bruise anyone's ego, or any institution's reputation, but to encourage the medical community to be open—disclose, take ownership and remedy mistakes forthrightly to everyone concerned. By being open, they can help others and themselves relieve pain and suffering in this small world in which we all live our short lives. It is for this reason abbreviated names and acronyms were used; they were necessary to preserve the authenticity of this story.

2012

END NOTES

P 8   1. Transcript of discovery, Jen, November 17, 1997.

P 41   2. Burst suppression syndrome: Final and fatal stage of status epilepticus

P 48   3. Shock Trauma Air Rescue Society

P 50   4. Names of the STARS team that brought Bobby and his parents from Montreal on July 15, 1994: Nurse Deborah Mears; Paramedic Mike Lamacchia and ER Physician Dr. Lance Shepherd.

P 64   5. Myoclonus Status after Cardiac Arrest, Abstracts and Commentary, Neurology Alert, May 1994, pp. 67-69; Source: Wijdicks, E., et al.: Prognostic Value of Myoclonus Status in Comatose Survivors of Cardiac Arrest. Ann Neurology 1994; 35: 239–243.

P 65   6. Employee Assistance Program

P 69   7. PVS: persistent vegetative state

P 70   8. Tachycardia: rapid heart rate, as after exercise

P 82   9. MRI report

P 89   10. Bobby's deposition, December 22, 1997

P 91   11. Montreal police report 94-7-14

P 97   12. Neuropsychological testing assesses cognitive and behavioral manifestations of brain malfunction. The tests usually involve question-and-answer pencil-and-paper tests and constructional tasks.

P 98   13. Narrative Summary for Patient #0 87 74 46

P 102   14. The Canadian Resident Matching Service (CaRMS) Corporation works in close cooperation with medical schools and students to provide a computer match for entry into postgraduate medical training.

15. *Calgary Herald* June 5, 1989, "Examples of Terry Fox inspires next generation" by Eleja Ross
P 104   16. Bobby's deposition, December 22, 1997
P 113   17. Kathleen E. Norman, B.Sc.P.T., pht 95803 (PhD candidate, Rehabilitation Science, McGill University) physiotherapist, L'Esprit-Sport Rehabilitation: "During the coma, he (Bobby) went into status epilepticus, and it took several days for the brain seizures to be appropriately controlled." "The neuronal damage has resulted in a constellation of problems in his coordination of movement. These coordination problems affect both movements at a fine level as well as movements involving the whole body."
P 115   18. Dr. Wilder Penfield, first director of the MNI, neurosurgeon, pioneered in surgical treatment of epilepsy, author of *No Man Alone*
P 116   19. Local community service center, Montreal
20. Medical (handicap) transport and Société de transport de Montréal
P 128   21. "MD sues over treatment, $4.4-million suit in case of peanut allergy reaction," *Calgary Herald*, July 12, 1995.
P 184   22. Accessible transit service for persons with physical disabilities
P 206   23. Canadian Charter of Rights and Freedoms
The Charter brings us together and celebrates our diversity. It protects the many rights and freedoms that make Canada a just society. Here are some of them:
    Freedom of expression
    Freedom of conscience and religion
    Freedom to gather in peaceful groups
    The right to live free from discrimination
    The right to receive services from the Government of Canada in English or French
    The right to vote and run for office
    The right to live and work anywhere in Canada

> The Charter reflects the pride of Canadians in the multicultural fabric of our society. It protects the rights of women, Aboriginal people and minority language groups.

P 224   24. Oil–water separator developed by the American Petroleum Institute to process refinery waste water

P 258   25. High-occupancy vehicle lane reserved for more than one occupant in a car

ABBREVIATIONS

ABMS	American Board of Medical Specialties
ABG	arterial blood gas
ABP	average (of systolic and diastolic) blood pressure
BJV	Bennett Jones Verchere
BP	blood pressure
CaRMS	Canadian Resident Matching Service
CCRF	Canadian Charter of Rights and Freedoms
CGH	Calgary General Hospital
CLSC	Centre local de services communautaires (local community service centre)
CMPA	Canadian Medical Protective Association
CPR	cardiopulmonary resuscitation
CRA	cardiorespiratory arrest
CRHA	Calgary Regional Health Authority
CAT	computerized axial tomography (also known as CT Scan)
DC	discontinue
EAP	employee assistance program
EEG	electroencephalogram
EQ	emotional intelligence ("quotient")
ER	emergency room
ET	endotracheal
HOV	high-occupancy vehicle (lane)
ICU	intensive care unit
IV	intravenous
JDR	judicial dispute resolution
LPH	Lakehead Psychiatric Hospital
MNI	Montreal Neurological Institute

MRI	magnetic resonance imaging
NG	nasogastric
NPH	Novolin N, Humulin N (insulin)
NR	nonresponsive
Pt	patient
PVC	premature ventricular contractions
PVS	persistent vegetative state
QC	Queen's Counsel
REM	rapid eye movement
RN	registered nurse
SOC	statement of claim
STCUM	société de transport de Montréal (public transit system)

LIST OF PEOPLE

Adolfo: narrator's colleague
Al: Jen's father
Albert: patient; Calgary businessman who aspirated and became severely impaired
Alfonso: homecare worker from the CLSC
Alice: Mon's classmate's mother
Allen: lawyer
Allison: department secretary, LPH
Andrew: neurology resident, Ottawa General Hospital
Annagret Rinaldi: court reporter
Annette: lawyer in Montreal
Barb: Nan's sister
Beatrice: ICU/ER nurse who became a malpractice lawyer (Montreal)
Bill: lawyer, hired (Calgary)
Bobby: son, 22 in 1994
Boni: secretary, review course, Ottawa
Brenda: worked in JGH accounting department
Brian: malpractice lawyer (Calgary) who filed the lawsuit and then dropped out
Bruce: old orderly
Buffy: caregiver from Spectrum Health Care agency
Carroll: Bill's secretary
Cheryl: narrator's secretary
Cheryl: nurse, FHH
Cheryl: Bobby's friend from California
Chris: Bill's secretary
Christine Egner: ICU nurse, JGH

Constable Benoit: CUM
Constable Masse: CUM
Criminal lawyer: referred by lawyer friend of Ratna's
Darryl: caregiver Toronto
Dan: Bobby's med school classmate
Denise: nurse, JGH
Donald: appendage lawyer
Doreen: lawyer in Edmonton
Dorothy Joudrie: celebrity socialite who nearly killed her husband, Earl
Dr. Anderman: Bobby's neurologist in Montreal
Dr. Jack Antel: chair of the MNI neurology program
Dr. Aubé: neurologist, MNI
Dr. Barton: physiatrist, CGH
Dr. Bern: neurology resident, FHH
Dr. Cohe: year 1-resident, JGH ICU
Dr. Collin: neurologist, MNI
Dr. Crow: second in command in the ICU, JGH
Dr. Cuttrell: PGY1 coordinator, McGill University Medical Residency program
Dr. Field: FHH
Dr. Demchuck: CGH
Dr. DeM: JGH
Dr. Doi: FHH
Dr. Francis: program director, MNI
Dr. Friedman: third-year internal medicine resident, JGH
Dr. Gordon: Bobby's neurologist
Dr. Gord: ICU fellow, JGH
Dr. Gra: ER, JGH
Dr. Jordan: expert
Dr. Kennedy: allergy specialist with privileges at CGH
Dr. Kimberly: anesthesiologist, FHH
Dr. Kinsella: director of bioethics, FHH
Dr. Koh: ER doctor, JGH

Dr. Lee: neurologist, FHH
Dr. M. Lee: neurologist, FHH
Dr. Leonard: neuropsychologist, MNI
Dr. Mitchell: Mt. Sinai
Dr. McGovern: physiatrist, doctor of physical medicine, CGH
Dr. Mukherjee: independent neurologist, FHH
Dr. Panis: neurologist, JGH
Dr. Powell: from STARS
Dr. Rose: ER doctor, JGH
Dr. Sand: ICU chief, FHH
Dr. Scho: neurologist, JGH
Dr. Scott: 1st-year neurology resident, FHH
Dr. Seshia: neurologist and specialist in coma
Dr. Sevick: radiologist, FHH
Dr. Shepard: on air ambulance
Dr. Dean Smith: dean of the faculty of medicine (Calgary)
Dr. Spa: director of ICU, JGH
Dr. Sull: ICU resident, JGH
Dr. Wolfram Tetzlaff: Bobby's old supervisor; Health Sciences laboratories
Dr. Samuel (Sam) Weiss: brain researcher in Health Sciences laboratories
Dr. Zac: staff neurologist, FHH
Dr. Zan: ICU chief, JGH
Edith: physio rehab therapist, Royal Victoria Hospital, Montreal
Elaine: Ratna's research assistant
Elaine: elderly volunteer, JGH
Elizabeth Robinson: court reporter
Ellen: ethics committee member, Health Sciences
Eric: homecare worker from the CLSC
Ethan: son of Gale's friend
Fay: nurse, JGH
Fay: building superintendant (Toronto)
Galag: BJV lawyer

Gale: narrator's wife
Gene: ward nurse; director of nursing, FHH
George: roommate, CGH
Gordon: malpractice lawyer (Montreal)
Grub: Virg's junior lawyer
Gupta: family friend
Helen: old friend of Bobby's
Helen: psych nurse
Ian St. John: homecare worker from the McGill University office of students with disabilities
Jackie: nurse, FHH
Jamie: law school graduate; greeter at law office, Calgary
Janice: nurse, FHH
JC: advisor with Nesbitt Burns
Jean-Pierre: lawyer (Montreal East)
Jen: Bobby's girlfriend
Jen's best friend: name was also Jen
Jessica: med student; daughter of a patient at FHH; friend of Mon
Jim: lawyer, Calgary
Joan: nurse, JGH
Joan: caregiver, Calgary
Joan: Bill's secretary
John: roommate, CGH
John: senior officer of the CRHA
Joseph (Joe): caregiver (Toronto)
Karen: Bobby's classmate
Kathleen: neurophysiotherapist and PhD candidate in Rehabilitation Sciences, McGill
Katrina: nurse, JGH
Keith: patient, CGH; became friends with Bobby
Ken: caregiver (Toronto)
Ken: lawyer, JGH
Kesh: homecare provider from Spectrum agency (Toronto)

Koshif: Bobby's high school friend
Krista: psychiatry resident at the Clarke Institute of Psychiatry, Toronto
Laura: nurse, FHH
Laurie: psychologist from interpersonal therapy clinic
Lawyer: friend of Ratna's
Liette: occupational therapist from CLSC (Montreal)
Linda: swim instructor, the Y, Calgary
Liz: also anaphylactic
Louis: from Lifeline (Montreal)
Louise: lead CRHA lawyer, for FHH
Maggie: attending nurse, FHH
Marc: co-counsel, Quebec City (son of anesthesiologist)
Marcel: anesthesiologist; father of Marc
Marg: unit's head nurse, FHH
Marg Haynes: social psychologist and faith-touch healer
Marge: patient care manager, FHH
Margit: Ethan's wife
Marnie: Bill's secretary
Marnie: private detective employed by Backtrack
Mart: defence counsel; lead CMPA lawyer
Michael: ethics committee member, Health Sciences
Molly: wife of ICU patient, JGH
Mon: daughter, 19 in 1994
Nan: Jen's mother; psychiatrist; divorced
Natalie: nurse, JGH
Neilly: son, 12 in 1994
Nihar: Grandmother ("Gramma")
Norah: lead JGH lawyer
Pastor Perry: wrote note in Bobby's chart, JGH, advice from Nan
Pat: nurse in charge, FHH
Pat: University of Montreal law department
Patty: accountant
Peter: Bobby's high school friend

Quigley: counsel for Dr. Sand
Ratna: Gupta's sister-in-law
Richard: appendage lawyer
Roon: Jen's lawyer
Russ Kelly: EAP counselor
Sagan: FHH
Sam: Mon's classmate's father
Sandra: social worker, FHH
Sergeant Richard Robert: from investigation branch of the CUM
Steve: roommate, CGH
Supriya: Calgary medical resident
Susan: ICU nurse, FHH
Susan: Bill's secretary
Trev: new-hire, co-counsel to replace Marc
Valeara Gordon: court reporter
Vij: Ratna's husband
Virg: lawyer
Wendy: young resident, FHH
Wishert: Ratna's grad student
Zia: FHH

ACKNOWLEDGEMENT

This manuscript was a massive block of words back in 2002. It needed shape, and shape it got through years of work, with assistance and advice from many: Lorna MacPhee, Paul Quarrington, Linda Pruessen, Antanas Sileika, Kim Moritsugu, John Metcalf, Kathleen Fraser, Maria Jelinek, Isobel Warren, Sharon Shore and Sherry Hinman, to name a few. They helped transform this old engineer into a writer, to tell the story of medical maladies—a life-lesson destined to die if it is not available to the general public. The historic digital revolution of the publishing industry has made publishing this book possible.

ABOUT THE AUTHOR

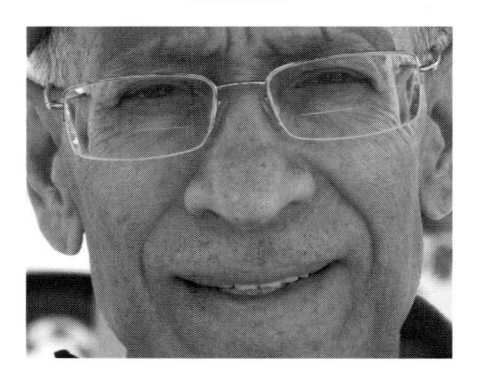

Prad Mitra Chaudhuri holds a master's degree in chemical engineering from the University of Windsor. Over the years, he has published many articles in recognized journals, and many papers internally for organizations that he worked for.

Following a life-changing event for him, and a life-altering event for the eldest of his three children, Prad turned his attention to preventable medical mistakes that affect numerous lives worldwide and cost healthcare systems enormous amount of money—money that should be used for diagnostic improvements and improvements in standards of care. He is affiliated with several engineering organizations—PEO, AIChE, CIC/CSChE—and writer's organizations—WEN, WCDR. He received creative writing and book publishing training at the Humber School of Creative & Performing Arts in Toronto, and at community-based writer's organizations.